LOW-IMPACT CARDIO WORKOUT FOR SENIORS

Safe and Soothing Cardio for Active Aging

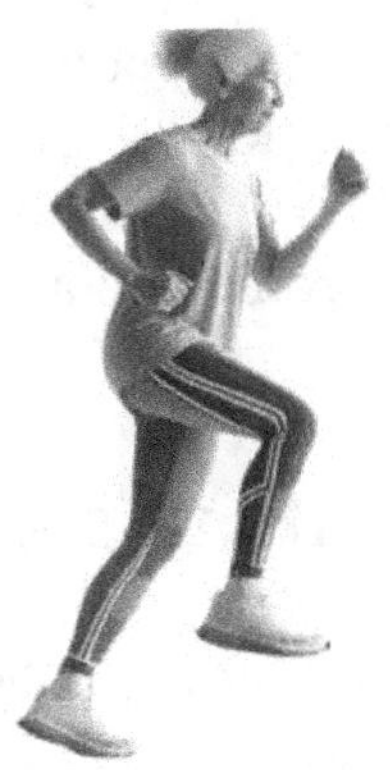

By Desmond T. Hall

Copyright © 2024 by Desmond T. Hall

Declaimer

This book is a work of nonfiction. Names, characters, places, and incidents are either the product of the author's imagination or are used fictitiously. Any resemblance to actual persons, living or dead, business establishments, events, or locales is entirely coincidental.

Other Books By this Author

Scan the QR Code Below to Get Access

TABLE OF CONTENTS

INTRODUCTION

Welcome to "Low-Impact Cardio Workout for Seniors," a guide designed to introduce seniors to the world of fitness in a way that is safe, pleasurable, and extremely helpful to both physical and mental health. As we age, being active becomes more important than ever, not only for our health but also for improving our quality of life. This book is intended to accompany you on a road to a more active, bright, and healthy living with low-impact aerobic activities created exclusively for seniors.

Low-impact cardio activities are mild on the joints, making them an excellent alternative for anyone seeking a workout that reduces stress on the body while yet giving all of the advantages of cardiovascular activity. These advantages include better heart health, greater strength and mobility, enhanced balance and coordination, and a lower chance of chronic illnesses. Furthermore, regular physical exercise can improve your mood, increase your energy, and help you keep your independence as you become older.

However, starting a new fitness adventure can be intimidating, especially if you're unclear where to begin or worried about injury. That is where this guide comes in. "Low-Impact Cardio Workout for Seniors" is designed to address these issues by providing precise instructions, safety advice, and motivating insights to guarantee that your fitness journey is both successful and sustainable.

We'll start by explaining what low-impact cardio is and why it's especially useful for seniors. You will learn about the many types of low-impact workouts and how they benefit your overall health. This book is designed to progressively expose you to different workouts, beginning with the most basic and foundational exercises and advancing to more complex routines. Each workout is supported by detailed directions, images, and modification suggestions to accommodate all fitness levels and physical restrictions.

Safety is a top priority, so we've dedicated an entire section to getting started properly. We'll go over fundamental pre-workout preparations, such as how to properly warm up and cool down, identify your body's signals to avoid injury and exercise safely.

Nutrition and hydration are critical components in supporting your fitness objectives, so we've given detailed instructions on how to properly nourish your body and keep hydrated. Understanding these concepts can help you get the most out of your workouts and stay energized.

Staying motivated may be difficult, especially when progress seems slow or life's difficulties get in the way. We'll discuss how to make reasonable, attainable objectives and find the desire to persist with your workout regimen over time. You'll also uncover inspiring stories from seniors who have altered their lives with low-impact cardio, demonstrating that it's never too late to begin and reap the advantages of an active lifestyle.

Our objective with this book is not just to give you a set of exercises, but also to inspire you to adopt a more active lifestyle that benefits your health and happiness. Whether you're just starting out in fitness or seeking to add new features to your current regimen, "Low-Impact Cardio Workout for Seniors" will help you every step of the way. Let us go on this road together, to a future full of strength, energy, and joy.

CHAPTER 1

What is Low-Impact Cardio?

Low-impact cardio is a type of cardiovascular exercise that reduces stress on the joints, making it a good choice for people who prefer a more delicate approach to physical activity. This sort of exercise raises the heart rate and enhances cardiovascular health while being gentler on the body's structural components, including the knees, hips, and back. It's especially useful for elderly, people just starting out in fitness, and those recuperating from an accident. In this portion of "Low-Impact Cardio for Seniors," we will look at the definition of low-impact cardio, its importance, and why it is a popular choice for staying active in one's later years.

Low-impact cardio is distinguished by the requirement for at least one foot to be in constant touch with the ground or equipment. This essential attribute considerably minimizes the amount of force exerted on the body when compared to high-impact exercises like as sprinting or leaping, in which both feet leave the ground and land with jarring force on the joints. Low-impact cardio provides for a continuous workout that improves heart health and endurance while reducing the chance of damage or strain on the musculoskeletal system.

Low-impact cardio consists of a number of workouts that may be modified to accommodate any fitness level or physical condition. Walking, cycling, swimming, and utilizing elliptical machines are all good examples of low-impact activities that may boost the heart rate and engage different muscle groups. Furthermore, flexibility and strength activities like yoga and Pilates can supplement low-impact cardiovascular workouts by improving balance, core strength, and overall physical performance.

Low-impact cardio is extremely beneficial to seniors' health. It is essential for treating and avoiding chronic diseases such as heart disease, diabetes, and osteoporosis since it improves cardiovascular health, regulates weight, and increases muscle and bone strength. Furthermore, frequent low-impact exercise can improve mental health by lowering symptoms of anxiety and sadness and increasing feelings of well-being. It also improves mobility and balance, both of which are essential for avoiding falls, which are a significant issue among the elderly.

Incorporating low-impact cardio into a senior's workout program can also help to enhance quality of life. It promotes independence by allowing older persons to carry out everyday tasks more effectively and with less weariness. Exercise also has social advantages when done in groups, such as courses or walking clubs, since it allows for social connection and community participation.

To get started with low-impact cardio, find activities that you love and can maintain over time. Begin with shorter, more manageable workouts, gradually increasing the length and intensity as your fitness improves. Always listen to your body and consult a healthcare physician or fitness professional to verify that the activities you choose are safe and appropriate for your health and fitness level.

Why Low-Impact Cardio is Ideal for Seniors

Low-impact cardio is especially beneficial for seniors, as it provides a safe and effective approach to stay active, improve health, and improve quality of life. Our bodies endure a variety of changes as we age, which can have an impact on our mobility, balance, and physical resilience.

These changes include decreasing bone density, muscle mass, and a greater risk of joint discomfort and injury. High-impact workouts, which place a lot of stress on the bones and joints, may worsen these problems, thus low-impact cardio is a better option for older folks.

One of the key reasons low-impact cardio is appropriate for seniors is its soft effect on the body. Walking, swimming, cycling, and utilizing elliptical machines are all low-impact exercises that provide the cardiovascular advantages required to maintain heart health and avoid chronic illnesses. This gentleness allows elders to engage in regular physical activity without concern of discomfort or injury that might result from more strenuous, high-impact exercises.

Furthermore, low-impact cardio may be readily tailored to the individual's fitness level and physical capabilities. Many low-impact workouts include variants and adaptations that allow you to raise or reduce the intensity without stressing your body. This versatility allows seniors to begin at a comfortable level and progressively increase their endurance and strength over time, which contributes to a consistent exercise regimen.

Low-impact cardio also helps seniors improve their balance and flexibility, which is a huge advantage. These exercises frequently involve numerous muscle groups and need coordination, which can help lower the risk of falls, a significant worry among older persons. Seniors may improve their balance and stability by strengthening their muscles and increasing joint mobility, all of which are essential for completing everyday activities safely and independently.

Low-impact cardio has significant mental and emotional advantages. Regular physical activity has been demonstrated to alleviate depression and anxiety symptoms, boost mood, and improve cognitive performance. Staying active with low-impact cardio can help elders improve their mental health and overall well-being. It encourages social engagement, particularly in group classes or activities, which contributes to a happy mental state.

Low-impact exercise can help seniors control their weight and battle the impacts of obesity and other illnesses like type 2 diabetes and high blood pressure. Seniors who maintain a healthy weight can minimize the strain on their joints, increase mobility, and lower their chance of developing chronic health problems.

Low-impact cardio can help seniors gain more energy and independence. The activities increase endurance and stamina, helping older persons to complete everyday duties more efficiently and without tiredness. This enhanced skill can significantly improve a senior's ability to live independently and have a greater quality of life.

How to Use This Book

This book, "Low-Impact Cardio Workout for Seniors," is intended to serve as a thorough guide to assisting seniors in safely and successfully engaging in physical exercise that improves their health without placing excessive strain on their bodies. To get the most out of this book, adopt the following approach:

Begin with Understanding.

Start by reading the introductory parts, which explain what low-impact cardio is and why it's especially useful to seniors. A thorough comprehension of these concepts will allow you to recognize the significance of each activity as well as the necessary safety precautions.

Assess Your Current Fitness Level

Before you begin the activities, examine your current fitness level. This evaluation will assist you in determining where to begin and, if necessary, whatever adaptations to the exercises are required to fit your talents and limits.

Follow the Exercises Step by Step.

The workout chapters are organized to take you through a variety of low-impact cardio routines, ranging from the most basic to the most sophisticated. Follow these procedures carefully, paying close attention to the directions and images to verify that you're doing each action properly and safely.

Incorporate Nutritional and Hydration Advice.

Do not skip the nutrition and hydration parts. These factors are critical for supporting your fitness goals and general well-being. To supplement your training program, follow the tips for healthy nutrition and staying hydrated.

Set realistic goals and monitor your progress.

Use the motivation and goal-setting chapters to help you develop reasonable, attainable exercise objectives. Tracking your progress may be extremely rewarding and encouraging, allowing you to stay dedicated to your fitness goals.

Stay Consistent and Patient

Consistency is crucial to reaping the advantages of low-impact exercise. Be patient with yourself, and don't be disheartened if progress appears sluggish. Remember that the objective is to improve your health and quality of life in a sustained way.

Following these criteria will make this book a great resource on your path to a better, more active lifestyle. Whether you're new to exercising or wanting to modify your existing program to better meet your requirements as a senior, this guide will help you every step of the way.

CHAPTER 2

Understanding the Benefits

Understanding the benefits of low-impact cardio is critical for seniors beginning their fitness journey. This type of exercise is not only accessible and safe for people of all fitness levels, but it also provides a slew of health advantages that may dramatically improve quality of life in one's senior years.

Physical Health Benefits:

Low-impact cardio activities are intended to raise heart rate and promote cardiovascular health without causing undue stress on the body. Regular involvement in these activities can aid in the management or prevention of chronic illnesses including hypertension, heart disease, and type 2 diabetes. Low-impact cardio improves blood circulation and heart function, ensuring that all parts of the body receive the oxygen and nutrients they require to perform properly.

Another big advantage is increased physical strength and endurance. Low-impact exercises train diverse muscle groups, increasing overall body strength without the danger of damage that comes with high-impact activities. This enhanced muscle strength promotes joint health and can help with symptoms of arthritis and other joint-related diseases.

Enhancing Mobility and Flexibility

For elders, preserving mobility and flexibility is critical. Low-impact cardio exercises frequently include motions that enhance range of motion and reduce joint stiffness. Enhanced flexibility and mobility are essential for carrying out everyday tasks, lowering the risk of falling, and retaining independence.

Weight Management

Regular low-impact exercise helps with weight management by burning calories and increasing metabolism. Weight control is critical for minimizing joint stress, lowering the risk of obesity-related disorders, and improving general health.

Mental and Emotional Health.

Low-impact cardio has several advantages, including improved mental and emotional wellness. Endorphins, often known as the body's natural mood lifters, are released during exercise and can help to alleviate sadness and anxiety symptoms. Furthermore, regular physical activity has been related to better sleep, higher cognitive performance, and a stronger sense of well-being.

Social Benefits:

Many low-impact cardio exercises may be done in a group context, such as classes or walking groups. These social connections can help to alleviate feelings of loneliness and isolation, fostering a sense of community and belonging. Engaging with peers adds inspiration and encouragement, making it easier to stick to a fitness plan.

Independence and Quality of Life.

Finally, the numerous advantages of low-impact cardio help to preserve and improve the quality of life for seniors. Individuals can lead more active, independent lives by enhancing their physical health, mobility, and mental well-being. The capacity to conduct everyday tasks with ease, participate in favorite pastimes, and fully engage in life's moments demonstrates the power of low-impact cardiac fitness maintenance.

The Impact on Mobility and Independence

Low-impact cardio has a significant influence on elders' mobility and independence. As people age, keeping mobility becomes increasingly important for retaining independence and having a high quality of life. Low-impact cardio activities are critical in this environment, providing a safe and effective strategy to improve physical function, lower the risk of falling, and increase autonomy.

Enhancing Mobility

Mobility, or the capacity to move freely and effortlessly, is required for many daily tasks, including housework, shopping, and socializing. Low-impact cardio workouts, such as walking, swimming, cycling, and tai chi, emphasize motions that raise heart rate while being mild on the joints. These activities promote joint range of motion, flexibility, and muscular strength, all of which are necessary for mobility.

Regular low-impact aerobics can significantly enhance endurance and stamina. Over time, seniors may find it easier to climb stairs, travel longer distances, and participate in activities that demand prolonged physical effort. Such gains are directly related to increased mobility, as the body becomes more capable of doing physical tasks without weariness.

Preserving Independence

The capacity to move without pain or discomfort is intimately related to an individual's degree of independence. Seniors who maintain a high level of physical fitness through low-impact cardio are more likely to be able to do daily tasks independently, such as personal care routines and household chores. This autonomy is important for self-esteem and mental health since it promotes a sense of accomplishment and control over one's life.

Furthermore, better mobility minimizes the danger of falls, which are a prevalent worry among the elderly and frequently result in injuries and loss of independence. Low-impact cardio workouts, which build muscles, improve balance, and coordination, can greatly reduce this risk. This preventative measure is especially important since keeping physical integrity is critical to living independently.

CHAPTER 3

Getting Started Safely

Starting any new workout routine, especially for seniors beginning on a low-impact cardio adventure, needs careful planning to maintain safety and avoid damage. The instructions below are intended to help seniors start their fitness routines safely, maximizing the advantages of low-impact cardio while reducing dangers.

Consult with healthcare providers.

Before beginning a new fitness regimen, seniors should contact with their healthcare providers. This stage guarantees that the workouts selected are safe and appropriate for their individual health problems and physical ability. A healthcare practitioner can provide tailored advise and may suggest changes or precautions depending on an individual's health profile.

Understand your body.

Recognizing and comprehending one's physical limitations is critical when beginning a new training plan. Seniors should be aware of any areas of concern, such as joint pain, balance challenges, or cardiovascular disease, and alter their exercise regimen appropriately. Recognizing indicators of effort is also critical; symptoms such as extreme weariness, dizziness, or discomfort should not be overlooked.

Start slowly.

Rushing into a new fitness routine might result in overexertion and injury. Seniors should begin carefully, with short periods of low-intensity exercise, gradually increasing the intensity and length as their fitness improves. This progressive approach helps the body to adjust to increased physical demands while minimizing strain.

Concentrate on warm-up and cool-down.

A safe workout regimen must include proper warm-up and cool-down times. Warming up with mild stretching or light walking for 5-10 minutes helps to prepare the muscles, joints, and cardiovascular system for more vigorous action, lowering the chance of injury. Similarly, cooling down with moderate stretching and gradual movements allows the body to return to a resting state, reducing muscular discomfort and stiffness.

Prioritize proper form and technique.

Learning and maintaining good form and technique throughout any exercise is critical for avoiding injuries and maximizing workout efficiency. Seniors should seek advice from fitness specialists or reputable sources to understand how to do each activity correctly. Attention to form becomes even more crucial since it helps reduce pressure on joints and muscles.

Use the appropriate equipment and attire.

Wearing supportive footwear and comfortable, breathable clothes can improve the safety and comfort of an exercise. Exercise equipment, such as stationary cycles or elliptical machines, should be adjusted to meet the user's body size and capabilities to avoid strain and increase exercise efficacy.

Stay hydrated and listen to your body.

Hydration is essential for a safe workout program. Seniors should drink water before, during, and after exercise to avoid dehydration, which can cause dizziness and other health difficulties. Listening to one's body is also key; if an activity causes pain or suffering, it's best to pause and reconsider.

There is a distinction between the natural discomfort of exercise and the pain that suggests a problem.

Create a supportive environment.

Low-impact cardio can be more motivating and safer when done in groups or with a partner. Having someone to share the experience with may make exercise more fun and add a sense of accountability. In addition, having someone nearby can provide fast aid in the event of a crisis or emergency.

Getting started safely with low-impact cardio requires making educated, conscious decisions that promote well-being. Following these rules allows seniors to begin on their fitness path with confidence, knowing that they are taking the essential precautions to preserve their health and maximize the rewards of their efforts.

Pre-Workout Preparation

Pre-workout preparation is an essential part of any exercise routine, especially for seniors beginning on a low-impact cardio adventure. These preparations guarantee that people are both physically and psychologically prepared to engage in physical exercise, lowering the risk of injury and enhancing the benefits of the workout. Here's a detailed guide to successful pre-workout routines for seniors.

Consultation with healthcare professionals.

The first step in pre-workout preparation is to speak with healthcare specialists. This is especially crucial for seniors who have pre-existing health concerns or who have never exercised before. A healthcare professional may provide vital insights into any precautions that should be taken, as well as advice on the best activities for particular health statuses and fitness objectives.

Setting Realistic Goals.

Before beginning any workout, it is critical to establish reasonable, attainable goals. Seniors' aims may include improving flexibility, cardiovascular health, muscle strength, or simply keeping an active lifestyle. Clear goals allow you to personalize your training to your unique demands while also providing incentive.

Understanding The Workout Plan

Before commencing your workout, familiarize yourself with the strategy to guarantee a smooth and safe session. It entails understanding the exercises included in the session, their sequence, and the proper approaches for doing them. This understanding aids in mental preparation for the workout and ensures that each exercise is completed safely and successfully.

Hydration and Nutrition

Before beginning an exercise, ensure that you are well hydrated. Drinking water before exercise prevents dehydration, which can cause weariness, dizziness, and other health problems. Eating a small, healthy supper or snack might also help you stay energized during your activity. To avoid pain, let plenty of time for digestion before beginning the workout.

Wearing appropriate attire

Wearing the appropriate clothes may have a big impact on the comfort and efficacy of your workout. Seniors should wear comfortable, breathable clothes that does not hinder movement. Supportive footwear is also essential, particularly for workouts that require walking or standing, to promote stability and prevent falls.

Warm-Up

A solid warm-up is one of the most crucial aspects of pre-workout preparation. Warm-up activities ease the body into physical activity by gradually boosting heart rate and blood flow to the muscles. A warm-up for seniors may consist of gentle walking, stretching, or mobility exercises. This not only helps to prevent injuries but also increases the overall efficacy of the activity.

Equipment and Environment Safety Check

Before beginning to use workout equipment, make sure that everything is properly and safely set up. This includes checking the settings of stationary cycles, treadmills, and elliptical equipment to ensure personal comfort and safety. Furthermore, keeping the training area clear of obstructions or dangers is critical to avoiding accidents and falls.

Mental Preparation

Finally, mental preparation is a sometimes forgotten part of pre-workout regimens. Approaching the gym with a positive attitude and reasonable expectations will help you stay motivated and focused, resulting in a more pleasurable and productive workout. Taking a few seconds to mentally prepare can also help seniors focus and fully participate in the impending physical activity.

By implementing these pre-workout preparations, seniors may safely and efficiently begin their low-impact cardio exercises, ensuring they are completely prepared to reach their fitness objectives while reducing their risk of injury.

Warm-Up Essentials

Warm-ups are an important part of any exercise routine, especially for seniors who do low-impact cardio activities. The fundamental purpose of a warm-up is to progressively prepare the body for more intensive physical exercise, hence improving performance and lowering the chance of injury. A comprehensive warm-up practice boosts blood flow to the muscles, elevates body temperature, and improves flexibility, which is especially important for seniors who want to protect their safety and get the most out of their activity.

Dynamic Stretching

Dynamic stretches are excellent for warming up because they include movement and gradually prepare the body for the range of motion necessary during activity. Examples include arm circles, leg swings, and modest walking lunges. These movements serve to release the joints, raise muscle temperature, and promote general mobility.

Light cardiovascular activity.

Begin with modest cardiovascular exercises like walking in place, leisurely riding on a stationary bike, or a gently row on a rowing machine to gradually boost your heart rate. This moderate increase in heart rate serves to prepare the cardiovascular system for the next activity, ensuring that the heart and lungs are ready to meet the body's increased need for oxygen during exercise.

Breathing Techniques

Incorporating breathing methods into the warm-up might also help. Deep, diaphragmatic breathing increases oxygen flow to the muscles while also promoting calm and focus, preparing both the mind and body for activity.

Warm-ups tailored to each individual

Seniors should adjust their warm-up exercises to their personal needs and the activities scheduled for their workout. The warm-up should imitate the motions of the next exercise at a lesser intensity to prepare the body for the workout's unique demands.

A well-structured warm-up is essential for seniors, laying the groundwork for a safe and productive low-impact cardio activity. Seniors may promote health and prevent injuries by including dynamic stretches, mild aerobic workouts, and correct breathing methods into their workout routines.

Understanding Your Body's Limits

Understanding your body's limits is an important component of any exercise plan, especially for seniors doing low-impact cardio routines. This information is essential for avoiding accidents, assuring the effectiveness of activities, and fostering long-term health and wellness. As we age, our bodies endure a variety of changes that may impair our physical capacities, making it even more critical to identify and respect these boundaries.

Recognize Physical Signals

Understanding your body's limits requires learning to identify the physical cues it sends. These symptoms may include shortness of breath, extreme weariness, muscular discomfort, or acute aches. While some discomfort is natural while engaging in physical exercise, especially for novices, pain is a strong indication that you should pause and reconsider. It's critical to distinguish between typical discomfort caused by activity and pain that indicates possible damage or injury.

Importance of Gradual Progress

Gradual improvement is essential in any workout plan. Sudden changes in exercise intensity or length might cause seniors to overexert themselves and sustain injuries. Instead, gradually increasing the intensity and duration of workouts enables the body to adjust safely. This method guarantees that you are challenging yourself without pushing your body past its limits, producing strength and endurance increases with minimal danger.

Listen to Your Body

Listening to your body is paying attention to its requirements and responding properly. This might include taking a day off if you're feeling extremely tired or altering activities to account for any discomfort or limits. Hydration, diet, and proper rest are also important aspects of listening to your body since they promote healing and general health.

Consultation with Healthcare Professionals

Regular check-ups with healthcare specialists can help elders understand their physical capabilities and limitations. Medical issues such as arthritis, osteoporosis, or heart disease may necessitate special changes to a fitness regimen. Healthcare practitioners may provide specific guidance to ensure that exercise regimens are safe and successful, taking into account any pre-existing health conditions.

The Importance of Rest and Recovery

Understanding your body's limits also entails acknowledging the significance of rest and rehabilitation. Adequate rest between workouts is vital for the body's healing and strengthening. Seniors may require more recovery time than younger people, emphasizing the importance of patience and providing enough time for the body to recover after exercise.

Safety During Exercise

Safety while exercise is critical, especially for seniors beginning a low-impact cardio plan. As the body ages, it becomes more prone to injury and longer to heal, making it critical to implement procedures that promote safety and reduce risk. Here are some important considerations for being safe when exercising, particularly for seniors doing low-impact cardio activities.

Understand and respect your physical limitations.

Recognizing and respecting your physical limitations is the first step toward exercising safely. This includes being aware of any pre-existing health disorders, such as heart or joint difficulties, and adapting your exercise intensity and duration accordingly. To avoid overexertion, start with activities that are appropriate for your current fitness level and gradually increase the intensity.

Use the proper equipment and attire.

Using the proper equipment and clothes can dramatically minimize the likelihood of accidents and injuries. To avoid slips and falls, you should choose supportive footwear with adequate grip and stability. Furthermore, utilizing any workout equipment appropriately, whether resistance bands, weights, or cardio machines, guarantees that activities are carried out safely.

Warm up and cool down.

A complete warm-up before exercising, followed by a cool-down, is critical for preparing the body for physical activity and avoiding muscular injuries. Warm-up exercises should gently raise your heart rate and relax your muscles, whereas cool-down activities should gradually drop your heart rate and stretch the muscles utilized throughout your workout.

Stay hydrated.

Hydration is essential for avoiding overheating and dehydration, which can result in dizziness, muscular cramps, and other health difficulties. Drinking water before, during, and after exercise helps you stay hydrated and promotes overall health.

Listen to your body.

Paying attention to how your body feels when exercising is critical. If you feel discomfort, dizziness, or severe weariness, stop immediately and rest. These symptoms may signal that you're pushing yourself too hard or that the workout isn't right for you.

Maintain proper form.

Maintaining appropriate form while exercise is crucial to avoiding injury. Incorrect form can put tension on muscles and joints, potentially causing injury. If you're unclear how to do an exercise correctly, get help from a fitness specialist.

Monitor your surroundings.

Make sure your workout area is safe and clear of obstructions that might cause trips and falls. Adequate illumination and a clean, clutter-free floor space are critical for preventing accidents.

Incorporate Rest Days.

Rest days are crucial components of any workout regimen, particularly for seniors. Allowing time for the body to recuperate lowers the danger of overuse injuries and guarantees that you can exercise safely in the long run.

By following these safety rules, seniors may reap the many advantages of low-impact cardiac exercise while lowering their chance of injury, resulting in a happy and healthy exercise experience.

Recognizing Warning Signs

Recognizing warning indicators during exercise is critical for seniors to protect their safety and well-being when doing low-impact cardio activities. Being aware of these indications can help you avoid potential health problems and injuries. Here are some important warning indications that should not be ignored:

- **Excessive fatigue.**

While it is natural to feel fatigued after physical exercise, severe exhaustion that does not correspond to the effort level may indicate that your body is being pushed too hard. It's critical to distinguish between normal exhaustion after an exercise and extreme fatigue, which might signal overexertion or dehydration.

- **Dizziness or lightheadedness**

Feeling dizzy or lightheaded during or after exercise may indicate dehydration, low blood pressure, or even cardiovascular problems. If you have these symptoms, cease exercising immediately and sit or lie down.

- **Chest pain or discomfort**

Any chest pain or discomfort, including tightness or pressure, while exercising is a major warning indication that should not be overlooked. These symptoms might signal a heart problem, necessitating rapid medical intervention.

- **Shortness of breath.**

While elevated breathing rates are common during aerobic activities, experiencing shortness of breath that seems unnatural or out of proportion to the activity level is a red flag. If breathing becomes difficult or painful, stop the activity and rest.

- **Sharp or sudden pain.**

Sharp, unexpected aches, particularly in the joints or muscles, may suggest an injury. Continuing to exercise despite intense pain can worsen injuries, resulting in prolonged healing periods.

- **Unusual or persistent symptoms**

Any odd or persistent symptoms during or after exercise, such as nausea, severe headache, or excessive muscular weakness, should be treated seriously. These might be indications of underlying health problems that require medical attention.

Recognizing and responding to these warning signals is critical for staying healthy and safe when exercising. Seniors should always listen to their bodies and seek medical attention if they suffer any unusual symptoms during low-impact cardio activities.

Injury Prevention Techniques

Injury prevention is an important part of any workout routine, especially for seniors who may be more prone to injuries owing to reduced bone density, muscular strength, and joint flexibility. Adopting appropriate injury prevention practices allows seniors to reap the advantages of low-impact cardio activities while reducing their chance of damage. Here are some major measures for injury prevention:

1. Gradual progression.

One of the most effective strategies to avoid injuries is to gradually increase the intensity and duration of your workouts. Jumping into vigorous sports too early can overload the body, resulting in strains and sprains. Seniors should begin with modest workouts and progressively progress as their endurance and strength increase.

2. Proper warm-up and cool-down.

A complete warm-up before beginning an exercise regimen is required to prepare the muscles and joints for physical action. Warm-up activities should gradually boost heart rate and blood flow to the muscles, lowering the likelihood of injury. Similarly, cooling down after exercise helps to gradually drop the pulse rate and stretch the muscles, reducing stiffness and pain.

3. Concentrate on form and technique.

Maintaining good form and technique when exercising is critical for injury prevention. Incorrect form can cause unnecessary stress on joints and muscles, resulting in injury. Seniors should seek coaching from fitness specialists to acquire proper exercise technique and check their form on a regular basis.

4. Use appropriate equipment.

Wearing supportive footwear and utilizing the proper workout equipment can dramatically lower the chance of injury. Shoes with enough cushioning and support protect the joints during exercise, while properly maintained equipment provides safe and successful exercises.

5. Listen to your body.

Paying attention to the body's cues is critical for avoiding injury. If a workout causes pain or discomfort, you should stop and rest. Ignoring discomfort might result in more serious damage. Seniors should also allow enough recuperation time between workouts to avoid overuse problems.

6. Stay hydrated and nourished.

Proper hydration and nutrition improve muscular function and recovery, lowering the likelihood of cramping and injury. Drinking enough of water before, during, and after workouts, as well as eating a balanced diet, helps to keep the body healthy and resilient.

7. Provide Strength and Flexibility Training.

Incorporating strength and flexibility exercises into your training program helps increase muscular strength, joint stability, and range of motion, all of which help to prevent injuries. Strength training protects the joints by supporting the muscles that surround them, whereas flexibility exercises increase mobility and lower the chance of muscle strains.

Seniors may enjoy the tremendous health advantages of low-impact cardio activities safely if they use these injury avoidance strategies. These measures not only reduce the chance of injury, but also help to make exercise more fun and sustainable.

Post-Workout Care

Post-workout care is an essential component of any exercise regimen, particularly for seniors who perform low-impact cardio workouts. Proper post-workout care can help you recover faster, avoid injuries, and feel better in general. Here are some important features of post-workout care designed for seniors:

1. Cool down properly.

A gradual cool-down period is essential following any workout to safely return the heart rate and blood pressure to resting values. Gentle stretching and slow-paced exercises, like as walking, can help with this process. Cooling down helps to lessen the accumulation of lactic acid in the muscles, reducing discomfort and stiffness.

2. Stretching.

Stretching activities during the cool-down period can help increase flexibility, range of motion, and circulation. Concentrate on stretches that target the key muscle groups engaged throughout your workout. Stretching should be slow and controlled, without bouncing, to prevent muscular tension. Holding each stretch for 15-30 seconds can help lengthen muscle fibers and increase flexibility.

3. Hydration.

Rehydrating after exercise is vital for replacing fluids lost via perspiration and breathing. Water is normally adequate for hydration, but in the case of prolonged or strenuous exercise, seniors may benefit from electrolyte beverages to replace salt and potassium stores. Staying hydrated promotes recovery and reduces dehydration.

4. Nutrition.

Consuming a balanced meal or snack after exercise can help with muscle repair and energy replacement. Meals should contain a mix of proteins for muscle repair and carbs for energy replenishment. Lean protein sources, healthy grains, fruits, and veggies are all potential ingredients for nutritious post-workout meals.

5. Rest and Recovery.

Adequate rest is necessary for the body to recover and strengthen itself following an exercise. Seniors should obtain proper sleep and allow plenty of time between workouts for muscular recuperation. Including rest days in your training plan can help avoid overuse injuries and improve performance in future exercises.

6. Track Your Body's Response

It is critical to monitor how the body responds in the hours and days after an exercise. Mild soreness is typical, but prolonged pain or discomfort might suggest overexertion or an injury. Seniors should be aware of their body's signals and adapt their exercise level or frequency accordingly.

7. Use recovery tools.

Using rehabilitation items like foam rollers or massage balls can assist relieve muscular tension and increase blood flow to the muscles. These items might be very useful for elders to relieve pain and increase mobility.

Seniors who prioritize post-workout care can get the most out of their low-impact cardio activities, recover faster, and preserve their health and mobility. This holistic approach offers a balanced and sustained training plan that promotes long-term health.

Cooling Down

Cooling down after low-impact aerobic activities is an important step for seniors since it promotes healing, increases flexibility, and helps prevent injuries. A effective cool-down regimen gradually lowers the pulse rate and relaxes the muscles, returning the body to a resting condition. This section discusses the necessity of cooling down and offers suggestions for successful cool-down procedures for seniors after low-impact aerobic activities.

Importance of Cooling Down

The cool-down phase assists the body in recovering from the stress of exercise by gradually reducing the heart rate and blood pressure, lowering the risk of dizziness and fainting following strenuous activity. It also helps to remove waste products from the muscles, including lactic acid, which can build up during physical exercise and lead to muscular discomfort and stiffness. Furthermore, cooling down can assist to lower the risk of muscular cramps and stiffness in the immediate post-exercise period, while also enhancing flexibility, which benefits in the long-term maintenance of muscle and joint health.

Components of an Effective Cooldown

- Gradual reduction of exercise intensity

Begin the cool-down phase by gradually lowering the intensity of your cardio workout. For example, if you've been walking quickly, slow down to a leisurely stroll for 5-10 minutes. This progressive decline allows the body to adapt seamlessly from an active to a more resting state.

- Stretching

After the first slow-down time, including stretching activities that target the key muscle groups engaged throughout your workout. Concentrate on static stretches, in which you lengthen the muscle to a point of modest tension and keep it there for 15-30 seconds. Stretching can increase flexibility, improve range of motion, and relieve muscular tension. Stretching the calves, hamstrings, quadriceps, and lower back is important since these muscles are frequently used during low-impact aerobic workouts.

Breathing Techniques

During the cool-down, use deep, regulated breathing to assist relax the body and lower your pulse rate. Deep breathing can also enhance oxygen flow to the muscles, promoting healing and relaxation.

Hydration

Replacing fluids lost during exercise is an important aspect of the cooling down process. Drinking water or an electrolyte-replenishing drink might help you stay hydrated and recover faster.

Mindfulness and Relaxation

The cool-down phase is an ideal time for mindfulness and relaxation techniques like moderate yoga positions or guided relaxation. These techniques can help to reduce stress, relax the mind, and improve general well-being.

Cool-down Exercises for Seniors

slow strolling: Begin to taper down your cardiac activity with a few minutes of slow strolling.

- Stretching: Perform static stretches with the goal of increasing muscular flexibility and relaxation.
- Tai Chi or Yoga motions: These smooth, flowing motions can assist to concentrate the mind and body, which aids with the cooling down process.

Cooling down is a crucial component of any fitness regimen, particularly for seniors. It allows for a safer transition to rest, reduces post-exercise soreness, and maximizes the health advantages of physical activity. Seniors may improve their entire exercise experience by including a deliberate and comprehensive cool-down into their workout routine, improving health, flexibility, and well-being as they age.

Stretching and Flexibility

Stretching and flexibility exercises are essential components of any complete fitness program, especially for seniors. These techniques not only improve range of motion and mobility, but also aid in injury prevention, muscle healing, and general physical comfort. As we age, our muscles and joints become less flexible, resulting in less mobility and a higher risk of injury. Stretching and flexibility exercises can be used into low-impact aerobic workouts to prevent age-related changes and improve senior quality of life.

The importance of stretching

Stretching entails gradually tugging the muscles to lengthen them, hence increasing suppleness and flexibility. Regular stretching can offer a number of benefits for seniors, including:

- Increased Range of Motion: Stretching lengthens muscles and increases joint range of motion, making daily tasks more efficient.
- damage Prevention: Flexible muscles are less vulnerable to damage. Stretching warms up the muscles before physical exercise, lowering the chance of strains and sprains.
- Stretching promotes muscle healing and can reduce discomfort after exercises by increasing blood flow and nutrition delivery to the muscles.

- Improved Posture and Balance: Flexibility exercises help address muscular imbalances and improve posture, which is essential for staying balanced and avoiding falls.

- Stretching can also help to relax the body and mind, lowering stress and tension.

Types of Stretching

Stretching techniques may be classified into numerous forms, each of which is effective for improving flexibility and range of motion.

- Static stretching is the practice of holding a stretch in a comfortable position for a certain amount of time, usually 15-30 seconds. This sort of stretching is most helpful when done after a workout during the cool-down period.

- Dynamic stretching involves regulated motions that prepare the muscles for action. Dynamic stretches, unlike static stretches, are performed without retaining a posture, making them great for warming up.

- Proprioceptive Neuromuscular Facilitation (PNF) is a more sophisticated stretching technique that combines both stretching and tightening the targeted muscle area. PNF stretching, which involves the aid of a partner or physical therapist, is extremely effective for building flexibility.

Introducing Stretching into a Senior's Routine

To reap the most advantages from stretching, seniors should integrate it into their daily routine, concentrating on main muscle areas such the neck, shoulders, chest, back, hips, thighs, and calves. Here are some tips for safe and efficient stretching:

- Warm up first: When your muscles are warm, they can stretch more readily. A brief stroll or a few minutes of mild activity can get the body ready for stretching.
- Concentrate on Breathing: Deep, calm breathing while stretching can boost the efficiency of each stretch and encourage relaxation.
- Avoid Pain: Stretching should never cause pain. To avoid harm, stretch only until you feel moderate tension, not pain.

- Consistency is key: Regular practice leads to increased flexibility. Incorporating stretching into your regular routine is essential for long-term benefits.

- Seek Professional Guidance: Seniors who are new to stretching or have special health problems should consult a fitness professional or physical therapist to verify that they are stretching safely and successfully.

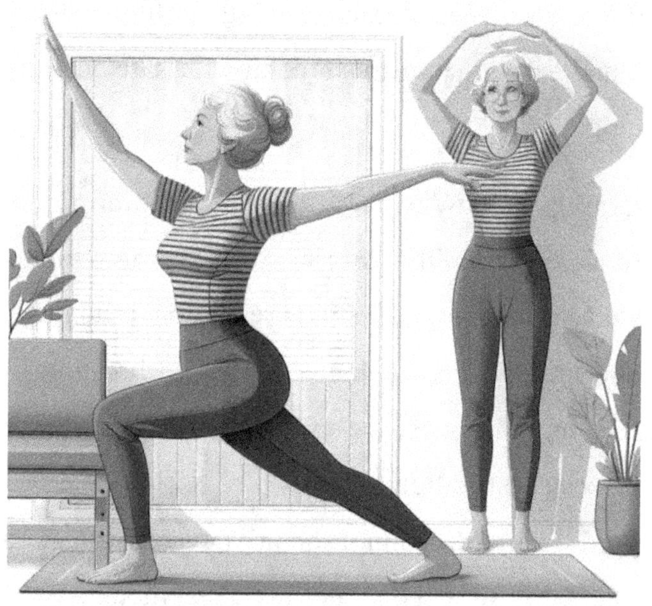

CHAPTER 4

Cardio Exercises Overview

Cardiovascular workouts, sometimes known as cardio, are intended to raise the heart rate and improve cardiovascular health. Low-impact cardio workouts are especially good for seniors since they reduce joint stress while still providing the many health benefits associated with regular physical activity. This review will look at numerous low-impact cardio activities ideal for seniors, highlighting their advantages and how to incorporate them into a fitness regimen.

Walking is a simple and effective low-impact cardio exercise for seniors. It does not require any extra equipment and can be modified to accommodate any fitness level. Regular brisk walking promotes heart health, strengthens bones, increases muscular power and endurance, and helps with weight control. Walking may be done outside in parks or on walking routes, or indoors in malls or on treadmills, making it a versatile exercise choice regardless of weather.

Swimming and water aerobics

Swimming and water aerobics are ideal activities for elderly. Water's buoyancy decreases joint impact, making these exercises appropriate for people who have arthritis or mobility concerns. Swimming works various muscle groups while improving cardiovascular health, flexibility, and muscle strength. Water aerobics sessions, which are typically tailored particularly for seniors, may also provide a social component, increasing motivation and enjoyment.

Cycling

Stationary cycling or outdoor biking on flat, level terrain can be an excellent low-impact cardio training for elders. Cycling improves heart health, leg strength, and joint mobility without the negative effects of other kinds of exercise. Stationary bikes also allow for easy resistance level adjustments, allowing seniors to gradually increase the intensity of their workouts as their fitness improves.

Elliptical trainers

Elliptical machines give a low-impact cardiovascular exercise similar to walking or jogging, but with less stress on the joints. These machines may be adjusted for various resistance levels, allowing seniors to tailor their exercises to their fitness levels. Elliptical training improves heart health, endurance, and balance, making it an excellent choice for seniors seeking to maintain an active lifestyle.

Tai Chi & Qi Gong

Tai Chi and Qi Gong are mild forms of exercise that involve slow, deliberate motions, deep breathing, and meditation. While they may not raise the heart rate as much as other cardio workouts, they do have distinct advantages, such as increased balance, flexibility, mental concentration, and stress relief. These exercises are especially good for seniors since they can be tailored to individual abilities and have been demonstrated to lower the risk of falls.

Dancing

Dancing is a fun and efficient technique to raise your heart rate. Many community centers and gyms provide dance courses for seniors, such as ballroom, line dancing, and Zumba Gold®. Dancing promotes cardiovascular health, coordination, balance, and muscle strength. It also includes a social component, allowing seniors to engage with others and experience a feeling of community.

Yoga

While not generally thought of as a cardio workout, certain kinds of yoga can give cardiovascular benefits by mixing fluid movements with breath training. Vinyasa or Flow Yoga raises the heart rate gradually, boosting circulation and flexibility while also lowering stress and promoting mental health.

Incorporating a range of these low-impact cardio exercises into a weekly practice can help seniors attain a well-rounded fitness regimen that includes cardiovascular health, muscle strength, flexibility, and mental wellness. Seniors who choose activities they like are more likely to stick with them and receive the long-term advantages of an active lifestyle.

Walking and Step Exercises

Walking and step movements stand out as crucial components of a low-impact cardio workout, particularly for seniors. These exercises are accessible, need little equipment, and may be modified to accommodate different fitness levels. Here's an in-depth guide to safely and efficiently adding walking and step exercises into a senior fitness program.

Walking: Step 1: Select appropriate gear.

- Choose supportive, comfortable footwear with a decent grip to avoid slips and falls.
- Dress in loose, breathable clothes appropriate for the weather circumstances.

Step 2: Warm up.

- Begin with a 5-minute warm-up that includes easy stretching or leisurely walking to prepare your muscles and joints for the exercise.

Step 3: Establish a Comfortable Pace.

- Begin walking at a pace that modestly raises your heart rate while yet allowing you to speak easily. This is commonly known as the "talk test" and is a reliable predictor of moderate intensity.

Step 4: Maintain good posture.

- Keep your head up, gazing forward, and your shoulders relaxed yet straight.
- Swing your arms normally, with a tiny bend at the elbow.

- Lightly engage your core muscles when walking.

Step 5: Gradually Increase the Duration.

- Begin with shorter walks, aiming for at least 10-15 minutes if you are just getting started.
- As your endurance increases, gradually increase your walking duration, with the goal of walking at least 30 minutes most days of the week.

Step 6: Cool down.

- Finish your stroll with a 5-minute slower-paced walk to reduce your heart rate.
- Stretch your legs, back, and arms next.

Step exercises

Step 1: Equipment Setup

- Choose a low-rise aerobic step platform. To guarantee safety, place it on a sturdy, non-slip surface.

Step 2: Warm up.

- Warm up with 5 minutes of mild cardio, such as walking in place or gentle marching.

Step 3: Basic Step-Up.

- Stand facing the step, feet hip-width apart.

- Step up onto the platform with your right foot, then follow with your left, ensuring that both feet are on the step.

- Step down with the right foot, then the left, returning to the starting position.

- Repeat the process, swapping the lead leg each time.

- Perform this exercise for 1-2 minutes, progressively increasing the time as your fitness increases.

Step 4: Side step.

- Stand with the step on your right side.

- Step up with your right foot, then bring your left foot to meet it on the platform.

- Step down to the left side of the step, first with your right foot, then with your left, before returning to the starting position.

- Repeat for 1-2 minutes, switching sides.

Step 5: Kneelifts.

- Perform a standard step-up, but when you elevate the first foot, lift the opposing knee towards your chest.
- Step down and repeat with the opposing leg, including the knee lift.
- Continue the exercise for 1-2 minutes.

Step 6: Cool down.

- After your step workout program, do a 5-minute cool-down, such as gradual strolling around the room.
- Finally, perform lower-body stretching movements, focusing on the calves, thighs, and hips.

Walking and step exercises provide seniors with a safe and effective technique to enhance their cardiovascular health, balance, and strength. Seniors may get the advantages of these activities while reducing their risk of injury by beginning cautiously, paying attention to form, and gradually increasing intensity and length.

Seated Exercises

Seated exercises are a wonderful choice for seniors looking for low-impact workouts that boost cardiovascular health, flexibility, and muscular strength without placing excessive strain on their joints. These exercises are especially useful for people who have mobility limitations or find standing exercises difficult. Here's a basic step-by-step method for practicing sitting workouts.

To march while seated, first find a stable chair.

- Sit on a firm chair without armrests, with your feet level on the floor. Sit up straight and use your core muscles.

Step 2: Start Marching.

- Lift your right knee as high as is comfortable, then lower it. Repeat with the left knee.
- Continue alternating legs to simulate a marching motion. Swing your arms opposite your legs to raise your heart rate.
- Perform this exercise for 1-2 minutes, progressively increasing the time as you gain endurance.

Seated Leg Extensions

Step 1: Sit properly.

- Sit in the same strong chair, feet flat on the ground, hands resting on the chair's sides for stability.

Step 2: Extend your leg.

- Extend one leg at a time, straightening it out in front of you as far as possible without locking your knee.

- Hold the extension for a few seconds, then slowly drop your leg back to its original position.

- Alternate legs, doing 10-15 extensions per leg.

Seated Arm Circles

Step One: Arm Positioning

- Sit erect in the chair and stretch your arms straight out to the sides, shoulder height.

Step 2: Perform Circles.

- Rotate your arms in small circles, progressively increasing the size of each circle.

- After 30 seconds, reverse the orientation of the circles.

- Continue for 1-2 minutes, emphasizing controlled motions.

Seated Rows

Step 1: Position your arms.

- Sit up straight, feet flat on the floor. Hold your arms out in front of you, palms facing each other.

Step 2: Row.

- Bend and draw your elbows back, pressing your shoulder blades together like you're rowing.
- Extend your arms back out.
- Perform 10-15 repetitions, concentrating on the action from your upper back and shoulders.

Seated Torso Twists

Step 1: Starting Position

- Sit up straight, feet level on the ground. Place your hands behind your head, elbows wide.

Step 2: Twist your torso.

- Gently twist your upper body to the right, as far as you feel comfortable. Return to the middle, then turn to the left.
- Maintain your hips and legs looking forward, ensuring that the action originates from your torso.

- Perform 10-15 twists to each side in a calm, controlled motion.

Cool down and stretch.

After finishing your sitting workouts, stretch for a few minutes. To relax and extend your muscles, try doing sitting hamstring stretches, chest openers, and neck stretches.

Seated exercises are a safe and effective option for elders to participate in physical activity, with an emphasis on increasing cardiovascular health, strength, and flexibility while reducing the risk of falls and joint stress. Seniors who incorporate these basic exercises into their daily fitness program can maintain and even improve their physical health and well-being.

Water Aerobics

Water aerobics is an ideal low-impact exercise for seniors, providing advantages such as enhanced cardiovascular health, muscle strength, and flexibility while putting less strain on the joints. Water's buoyancy supports the body, lowers the danger of falls and injuries, and allows for actions that would be impossible on land. Here's a basic step-by-step approach to water aerobics, perfect for seniors wishing to improve their fitness in a safe, friendly atmosphere.

Getting Started:

Step 1: Select the Right Facility.

- Find a nearby pool that provides senior-specific water aerobics courses or has a specialized water exercise space. Ensure that the facility is clean and well-maintained.

Step 2: Safety first.

- Wear water shoes to avoid sliding and protect your feet.
- Choose a depth that allows you to stand comfortably with water at breast level.
- To avoid falls, always enter and exit the pool with steps or a ladder.

Warm-Up

Step 1: Waterwalking

- Start with a 5-minute warm-up by strolling in the shallow end of the pool. Begin at a moderate pace and gradually progress to a fast walk.

- Maintain proper posture, with your back straight and shoulders relaxed.

Main Exercises

1. **Aqua Jogging**
   - Stand in water so deep that your feet do not touch the bottom, or stay in the shallow end for extra stability.
   - You may simulate jogging by moving your legs in a running manner. Use your arms like you would when jogging on land.
   - Continue for 5 to 10 minutes, changing the intensity as necessary.

2. **Leg Lifts.**
   - Stand close the pool wall for support if necessary.
   - Lift one leg to the side while maintaining it straight, and then drop it back down. Repeat for the opposite leg.
   - Repeat 10-15 times per leg, focusing on controlled motions.

3. **Arm Circles**

- With your arms underwater, stretch them to the sides to shoulder height.

- Rotate your arms in tiny circles, gradually increasing it bigger. After 30 seconds, reverse direction.

- Continue for 2-3 minutes with controlled motions.

4. **Water Squats.**

- Stand with your feet shoulder width apart.

- Lower yourself into a squat stance with your back straight and your knees behind your toes.

- Push yourself back up to a standing posture, taking advantage of the water's resistance.

- Perform 10-15 squats with calm, controlled motions.

5. **Flutter Kicks**

- Hold on to the pool's edge or a kickboard for support.

- Extend your legs behind you and make tiny, quick kicks.

- Continue for 2-3 minutes while maintaining your core engaged.

Cool down with gentle stretching: Spend the final 5-10 minutes of your practice with moderate stretches in the water. Focus on extending your arms, legs, and torso.

If required, use the pool wall or a noodle as support.

Water aerobics is a fun and efficient approach for seniors to engage in physical activity while also reaping the therapeutic advantages of being in water. Seniors may improve their health, increase their mobility, and enjoy the companionship of group exercise courses by performing these basic exercises in the supporting environment of the water.

Creating Your Routine

Developing a specific low-impact cardio regimen is critical for seniors who want to improve their health, preserve independence, and improve their quality of life. A well-structured program is tailored to each individual's fitness level, preferences, and health status, assuring safety and efficacy. Here's how elders may set up their own low-impact cardio routine:

Assess your current fitness level.

Step 1: Evaluate your current fitness level. Think about any current health concerns, your mobility, and any suggestions from healthcare specialists. This examination aids in adapting your routine to your unique needs, hence reducing the chance of harm.

Set clear, attainable goals.

Step 2: Determine what you hope to achieve with your fitness regimen. Goals might include improving cardiovascular health, boosting flexibility, and muscle strength, as well as stress reduction. Setting objectives allows you to create a concentrated routine that directs your efforts successfully.

Choose appropriate low-impact cardio exercises.

Step 3: Choose workouts that match your fitness level and goals. Include a variety of activities to keep the program interesting and address all elements of fitness. Walking, swimming, cycling, water aerobics, and senior-specific mild aerobic programs are all options. Diversifying your routine might also help prevent overuse injuries.

Plan Frequency and Duration.

Step 4: Determine how frequently and how long you will workout. Begin with shorter, more frequent sessions, aiming for at least 150 minutes of moderate-intensity aerobic activity per week, the recommended amount for seniors. Break it down into reasonable chunks, like 30 minutes every day, five days a week.

Include the warm-up and cool-down phases.

Step 5: Every workout should start with a warm-up and finish with a cool-down. Warm-ups might involve easy stretching or brief walking to get the body ready for workout. Cool-downs should gradually reduce heart rate and incorporate exercises to increase flexibility and prevent stiffness.

Step 6: Enhance your cardio regimen with strength and flexibility workouts. These are necessary for maintaining muscular mass, joint health, and balance. Exercises with modest weights, resistance bands, or bodyweight movements such as squats and sitting exercises can be useful.

Listen to your body.

Step 7: Pay attention to how your body reacts to the routine. If you're experiencing pain or discomfort, change the intensity, duration, or kind of exercise. Regularly examine your regimen and make changes as your fitness improves or your interests shift.

To stay motivated, establish modest, reachable targets, exercise with a friend, or participate in group sessions.

Tracking your progress may give you a feeling of success and motivate you to adhere to your regimen.

Step 9: Always emphasize safety. Use proper equipment, dress appropriately, and keep hydrated. To avoid falls, pay careful attention to the surfaces on which you exercise.

Seek professional advice.

Step 10: Consult a fitness professional or physical therapist, especially if you're just beginning out. They may give useful information, assist with workout changes, and verify that your regimen is safe and successful for your unique requirements.

Creating a specific low-impact cardio plan enables seniors to reap the advantages of physical exercise while staying within their body's restrictions. Seniors may achieve their exercise objectives, enhance their general health, and live a more active, meaningful lifestyle if they plan their program properly and update it periodically.

Personalizing Your Workout

Personalizing your workout is essential for developing an efficient, fun, and long-term fitness regimen, particularly for seniors. A personalized workout is tailored to an individual's health problems, fitness level, preferences, and objectives, ensuring that workouts are both safe and useful. Here's how seniors may customize their low-impact cardio workouts:

1. Evaluate your health and fitness level.

Begin by assessing your present health and physical condition. Consider any chronic illnesses, such as arthritis, diabetes, or heart disease, that may limit your ability to complete specific workouts. Understanding your starting place helps you choose appropriate activities and create realistic goals.

2. Define your fitness goals.

Determine what you want to achieve with your fitness program. Goals might include improving cardiovascular health, increasing flexibility, improving balance, or decreasing weight. Clear goals govern workout selection and progress tracking, allowing for modifications as needed.

3. Select appropriate exercises.

Choose low-impact cardio routines that are appropriate for your goals and entertaining to you. Walking, swimming, cycling, and tai chi are all wonderful alternatives for seniors, since they provide cardiovascular advantages without putting too much strain on their joints. Incorporating activities you like boosts your chances of adhering to your regimen.

4. Consider the Frequency, Intensity, Time, and Type (FITT principle).

Decide how frequently you will exercise. Starting with 3-5 days a week is good for the majority of seniors.

difficulty: Select the difficulty level for your workouts. Use the "talk test" to confirm you're working at a moderate level and can chat but not sing during the exercise.

Time: Determine the length of each workout session. Begin with shorter sessions and progressively work up to at least 150 minutes of moderate-intensity exercise every week.

Type: Change up the exercises to target different muscle areas, enhance overall fitness, and keep the workout interesting.

5. Combine flexibility and strength training. Combine your aerobic routines with flexibility and strength training activities. This comprehensive approach improves overall fitness, promotes muscle and joint health, and lowers the likelihood of injury. Yoga, Pilates, and mild resistance training are great complements to a senior's exercise routine.

6. Customize Exercises for Your Needs

Modify workouts to fit any physical restrictions or preferences. If you are concerned about your balance, use chairs, walls, or pool noodles as support. If you have joint problems, stick to workouts with little joint impact, such as swimming or using an elliptical machine.

7. Monitor your progress and adjust accordingly.

Keep track of your progress toward your fitness objectives. As you get fitter, you may need to change the intensity or diversity of your activities to keep pushing your body and making progress.

8. Listen to your body.

Pay close attention to how your body reacts during and after exercise. If you feel pain or discomfort, alter the workout or see a doctor. Rest days are essential for healing, especially if you're feeling tired or injured.

9. Seek professional guidance.

Consider speaking with fitness specialists that specialize in senior fitness. They may provide specialized guidance, provide suggestions for changes, and assist in developing a fitness plan that is tailored to your unique requirements and objectives.

Personalizing your workout guarantees that your fitness regimen is tailored to your specific health needs, talents, and interests. A personalized strategy for seniors not only emphasizes the health advantages of exercise, but also increases enjoyment and motivation, paving the path for a more active, healthier lifestyle.

Incorporating Equipment

Integrating equipment into a low-impact cardio workout can dramatically improve the efficacy, diversity, and pleasure of seniors' fitness routines. The correct equipment may increase resistance, improve balance, and bring new difficulties, making exercises more beneficial and entertaining. Here's how seniors may safely and efficiently include equipment in their low-impact cardio workouts:

1. Resistance Bands.

Functionality: Resistance bands are flexible instruments for adding resistance to workouts, strengthening muscles, and improving flexibility without using heavy weights.

Use bands to do arm curls, leg stretches, and chest presses. Begin with low-resistance bands and progress to increased resistance as your strength develops.

Benefits: Increases muscular strength, flexibility, and joint stability. Ideal for training particular muscle areas and adaptable to a range of fitness levels.

2. Hand Weights Incorporating hand weights or dumbbells into aerobic exercises can improve muscular strength and endurance through resistance training.

Incorporate modest hand weights with walking or sitting activities to increase the intensity of the workout. Start with modest weights (1-3 pounds) to reduce strain, then gradually raise the weight.

Benefits: Increases muscular strength, metabolic rate, and bone density, all of which are important for avoiding osteoporosis.

3. Ankle Weights: Add resistance to lower body motions for increased challenge and effectiveness.

Wear ankle weights during leg lifts, water aerobics, or sitting workouts to build resistance and strength.

Benefits: Increases leg strength, balance, and intensity of lower-body workouts without the need of sophisticated apparatus.

4. Stability Balls: Exercise balls are useful for core development, balance training, and improved posture.

How to Use: Use a stability ball as a seat while completing upper body workouts with hand weights or bands. To activate the abdominal muscles, use core strengthening activities such as sitting marches or mild ball twists.

Benefits: Increases core strength, improves balance and stability, and helps to maintain appropriate posture. Using the ball also promotes minor muscle modifications, which improves coordination.

5. Stationary Bicycles: Stationary bikes offer a low-impact cardiovascular workout that improves heart health and leg strength without straining joints.

How to Incorporate: Begin with short, easy workouts, gradually increasing time and resistance as fitness improves.

Benefits: Improves cardiovascular health, strengthens the lower body, and may be readily tailored to different fitness levels.

6. Functionality: Water noodles, kickboards, and aquatic dumbbells provide resistance for more strenuous water exercises.

Include, using kickboards for leg kicks, water noodles for balancing exercises, and aquatic dumbbells for arm-strengthening workouts in the pool.

Benefits: Increases the efficacy of water aerobics, builds muscular strength, and promotes joint health in a buoyant, low-impact setting.

Safety Tips for Using Equipment

- **Start slowly:** To minimize overexertion, use lower resistance or smaller weights.

- **Maintain proper form**. Use the equipment as suggested to avoid injuries and ensure that the workouts are successful.

- **Consult professionals:** To learn how to use any new equipment correctly, consult with a fitness instructor or physical therapist.

Incorporating equipment into low-impact cardio exercises allows seniors to change up their exercise regimen, push their bodies in new ways, and reach their fitness objectives safely and effectively. Seniors can get the multiple advantages of a well-rounded exercise plan by selecting and effectively using the appropriate equipment.

Progress Tracking and Adjustment

Progress tracking and correction are essential components of a successful exercise regimen, especially for seniors who participate in low-impact cardio activities. These techniques entail routinely analyzing exercise progress and making required modifications to the training plan in order to maintain increasing health and fitness levels.

To track progress, first set baseline measures for important fitness markers including endurance, strength, flexibility, and balance. This might include measuring how long you can walk without tiring, how many repetitions of a certain exercise you can do, or how far you can reach in a flexibility test.

Keep a Workout Journal: Document your daily activities, including the type of exercise, length, intensity, and any personal sentiments or challenges you encountered throughout the session. This notebook becomes an invaluable resource for identifying trends, improvements, and areas that require attention.

Wearable fitness trackers or apps may automatically record activity duration, heart rate, and calories burnt, allowing you to easily measure your progress over time.

Adjustment

Set a regular plan for reviewing your progress, such as every 4-6 weeks. Compare your current performance to your baselines to find areas for growth or where development has plateaued.

Adjust Goals: Based on your assessment, modify your fitness objectives to stay tough yet doable. This might include increasing the time or intensity of your workouts, incorporating new exercises, or concentrating on flexibility or balance.

Modify Workouts: If some workouts become too simple or no longer pleasant, replace them with other activities that are appropriate for your current fitness level and goals. Consulting with a fitness professional can bring new ideas while keeping your regimen safe and successful.

Seniors may stay motivated, overcome plateaus, and improve their health and fitness by measuring their progress methodically and making intelligent modifications to their training routines.

Progress Tracker Journal

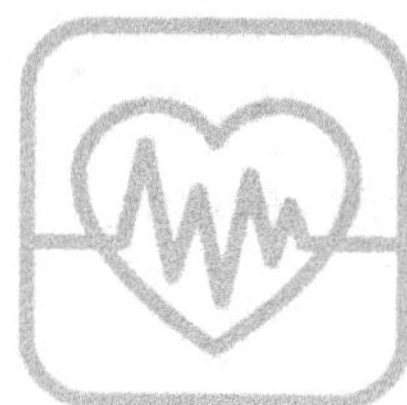

Cardio Workout Tracker

Week

Day

Monday Exercises:

Month

Weekly Goals

Tuesday Exercises:

Wednesday Exercises:

My Motivation

Thursday Exercises:

Friday Exercises:

Notes / Reminder

Saturday Exercises:

Sunday Exercises:

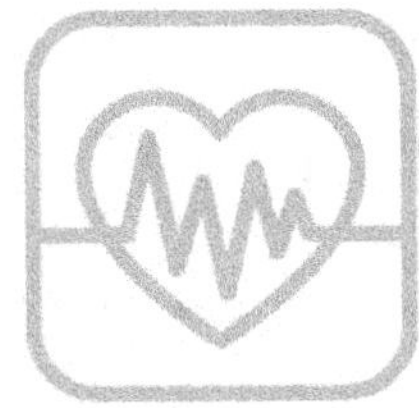

Cardio Workout Tracker

Week

Day

Month

Weekly Goals

Monday Exercises:

Tuesday Exercises:

Wednesday Exercises:

Thursday Exercises:

Friday Exercises:

Saturday Exercises:

Sunday Exercises:

My Motivation

Notes / Reminder

make
Yourself
. Proud .

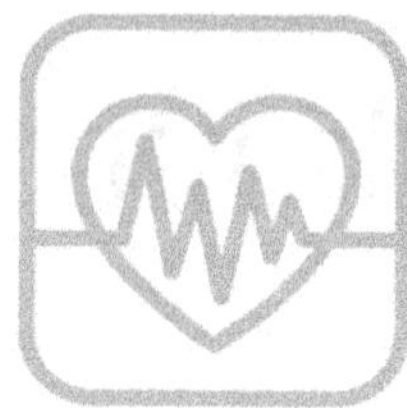

Cardio Workout Tracker

Week _______________________

Day _______________________

Month _______________________

Weekly Goals

Monday Exercises:

Tuesday Exercises:

Wednesday Exercises:

Thursday Exercises:

Friday Exercises:

Saturday Exercises:

Sunday Exercises:

- ● ☐ _______________________
- ● ☐ _______________________
- ● ☐ _______________________
- ● ☐ _______________________

My Motivation

Notes / Reminder

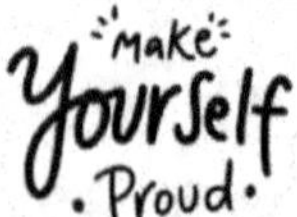

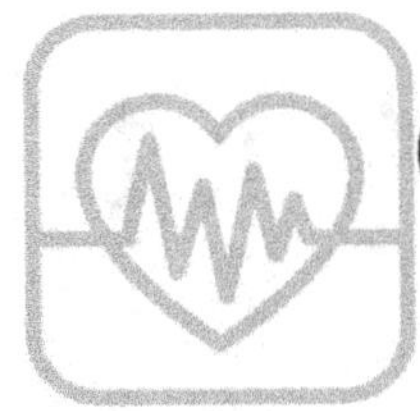

Cardio Workout Tracker

Week

____

Day

____

Month _______________________________

Weekly Goals

- ○ _______________________________
- ○ _______________________________
- ○ _______________________________
- ○ _______________________________

| Monday Exercises: |
| Tuesday Exercises: |
| Wednesday Exercises: |
| Thursday Exercises: |
| Friday Exercises: |
| Saturday Exercises: |
| Sunday Exercises: |

My Motivation

Notes / Reminder

make
Yourself
. Proud .

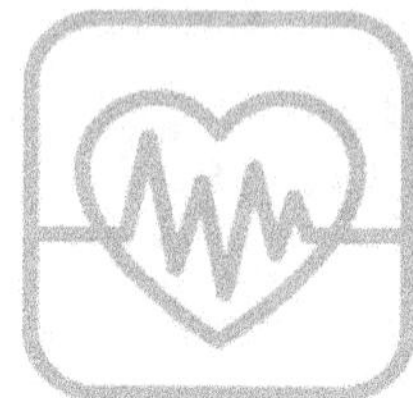

Cardio Workout Tracker

Week

Day

Month

Monday Exercises:

Weekly Goals

Tuesday Exercises:

Wednesday Exercises:

My Motivation

Thursday Exercises:

Friday Exercises:

Notes / Reminder

Saturday Exercises:

Sunday Exercises:

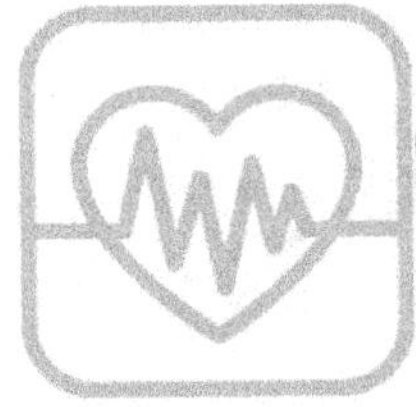

Cardio Workout Tracker

Week _______________________

Day _______________________

Month _______________________

Monday Exercises:

Tuesday Exercises:

Wednesday Exercises:

Thursday Exercises:

Friday Exercises:

Saturday Exercises:

Sunday Exercises:

Weekly Goals

- ☐ _______________________
- ☐ _______________________
- ☐ _______________________
- ☐ _______________________

My Motivation

Notes / Reminder

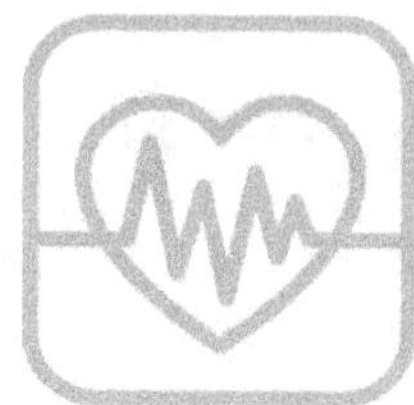

Cardio Workout Tracker

Week _______________________

Day _______________________

Month _______________________

Weekly Goals

- ○ _______________________
- ○ _______________________
- ○ _______________________
- ○ _______________________

Monday Exercises:

Tuesday Exercises:

Wednesday Exercises:

Thursday Exercises:

Friday Exercises:

Saturday Exercises:

Sunday Exercises:

My Motivation

Notes / Reminder

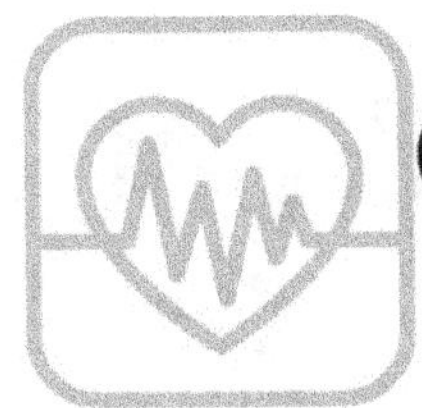

Cardio Workout Tracker

Week

Day

Month

Monday Exercises:

Tuesday Exercises:

Wednesday Exercises:

Thursday Exercises:

Friday Exercises:

Saturday Exercises:

Sunday Exercises:

Weekly Goals

My Motivation

Notes / Reminder

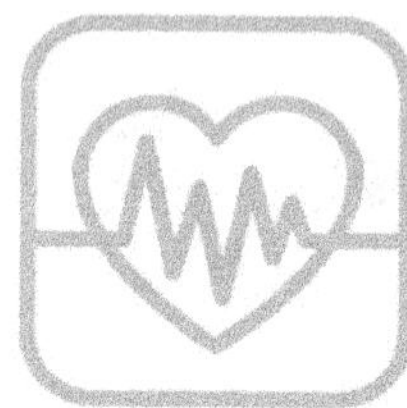

Cardio Workout Tracker

Week ________________________

Day ________________________

Month ________________________

Monday Exercises:

Tuesday Exercises:

Wednesday Exercises:

Thursday Exercises:

Friday Exercises:

Saturday Exercises:

Sunday Exercises:

Weekly Goals

- ⦿ ☐ ________________________
- ⦿ ☐ ________________________
- ⦿ ☐ ________________________
- ⦿ ☐ ________________________

My Motivation

Notes / Reminder

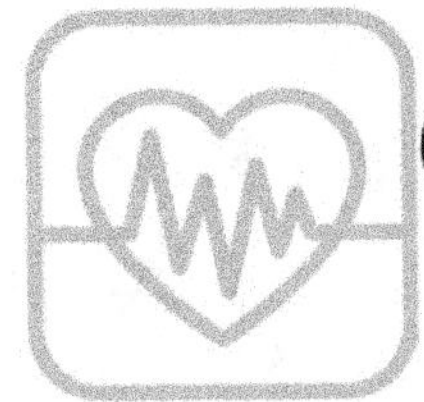

Cardio Workout Tracker

Week
____

Day
____

Month _______________________

Weekly Goals

- ☐ _______________________
- ☐ _______________________
- ☐ _______________________
- ☐ _______________________

Monday Exercises:

Tuesday Exercises:

Wednesday Exercises:

Thursday Exercises:

Friday Exercises:

Saturday Exercises:

Sunday Exercises:

My Motivation

Notes / Reminder

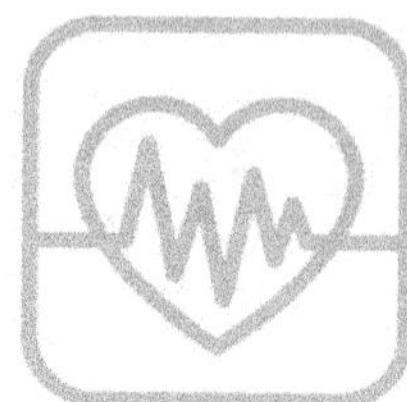

Cardio Workout Tracker

Week ______________________

Day ______________________

Month ______________________

Monday Exercises:

Tuesday Exercises:

Wednesday Exercises:

Thursday Exercises:

Friday Exercises:

Saturday Exercises:

Sunday Exercises:

Weekly Goals

- ○ ______________________
- ○ ______________________
- ○ ______________________
- ○ ______________________

My Motivation

Notes / Reminder

Make Yourself Proud

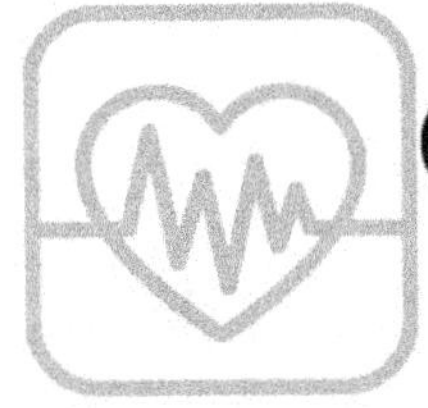

Cardio Workout Tracker

Week ________________________

Day ________________________

Month ________________________

Monday Exercises:

Tuesday Exercises:

Wednesday Exercises:

Thursday Exercises:

Friday Exercises:

Saturday Exercises:

Sunday Exercises:

Weekly Goals

- ☐ ________________________
- ☐ ________________________
- ☐ ________________________
- ☐ ________________________

My Motivation

Notes / Reminder

Make Yourself Proud

Setting Realistic Goals

Setting realistic objectives is an essential component of any successful fitness journey, especially for seniors starting low-impact cardio routines. Realistic objectives provide you direction, drive, and a sense of purpose, which makes your fitness journey more enjoyable and sustainable. Setting reasonable objectives is especially crucial for seniors, who may confront specific health difficulties and physical restrictions. It ensures safety, maintains motivation, and leads to long-term success. Here's how to develop realistic exercise objectives for seniors:

Understand your starting point.

Begin by examining your present physical condition, taking into account any health concerns, limits, and general fitness level. Understanding where you're starting from helps you establish tough but realistic objectives, reducing the chance of injury and disappointment.

Focus on health and well-being.

Goals should stress health and well-being over aesthetics or performance indicators, which may be irrelevant or unattainable for seniors. Goals may include improving cardiovascular health, increasing flexibility, improving balance, or reducing pain and stiffness, rather than obtaining a certain body weight or shape.

Make your goals specific.

Specific aims are more successful than vague goals like "get fit" or "be healthier". Instead, set specific, quantifiable objectives like "walk 30 minutes every day, five days a week" or "attend two water aerobics classes per week." Specific goals give a defined path and make it easy to monitor progress.

Ensure Goals are Achievable

While it is excellent to be ambitious, objectives should be achievable given your physical ability and lifestyle. Setting unrealistic objectives can lead to dissatisfaction and a lack of motivation if they are too tough to attain. Divide major goals into smaller, more attainable milestones to foster a sense of progress and accomplishment.

Keep your goals relevant.

Your exercise objectives should be consistent with your own interests, lifestyle, and health considerations. Goals that are significant and relevant to you are more inspiring and will be pursued. For example, if you prefer being outside, you may establish a goal to join a community walking club.

Set time-bound targets.

Including a deadline in your goals creates urgency and a feeling of direction. Time-bound goals, whether they include increasing endurance in three months or learning a new water aerobics routine in six weeks, promote consistency and dedication.

Write out your goals.

Documenting your objectives may help them become more tangible and act as a regular reminder of what you're working toward. Keep your written goals visible as a daily motivation.

Share your goals.

Sharing your objectives with family, friends, or other fitness lovers may give extra motivation and accountability. Knowing that others are aware of your goals might increase your motivation to achieve them.

Regularly review and adjust your fitness goals as you develop.

Throughout your trip, your talents and interests may evolve. Regularly examine your objectives to ensure they are both hard and attainable. If you see that particular goals have gotten too simple, consider raising their difficulty or creating new ambitions. If a goal becomes too lofty, alter it to better reflect your present fitness level and health situation.

Celebrate Achievements

Recognize and rejoice when you meet your goals, no matter how modest. Celebrating accomplishments reaffirms the importance of your work and encourages you to pursue other goals.

Be flexible and patient.

Fitness improvements, particularly for seniors, take time and constant commitment. Be patient with yourself and adapt your approach. If unanticipated health difficulties or other circumstances impede your progress, be prepared to adjust your goals accordingly.

Seniors may lay the groundwork for a low-impact cardio fitness plan by defining goals that are practical, detailed, achievable, relevant, and time-bound. This systematic approach not only promotes physical health but also improves mental well-being, resulting in a more active, meaningful lifestyle in the senior years.

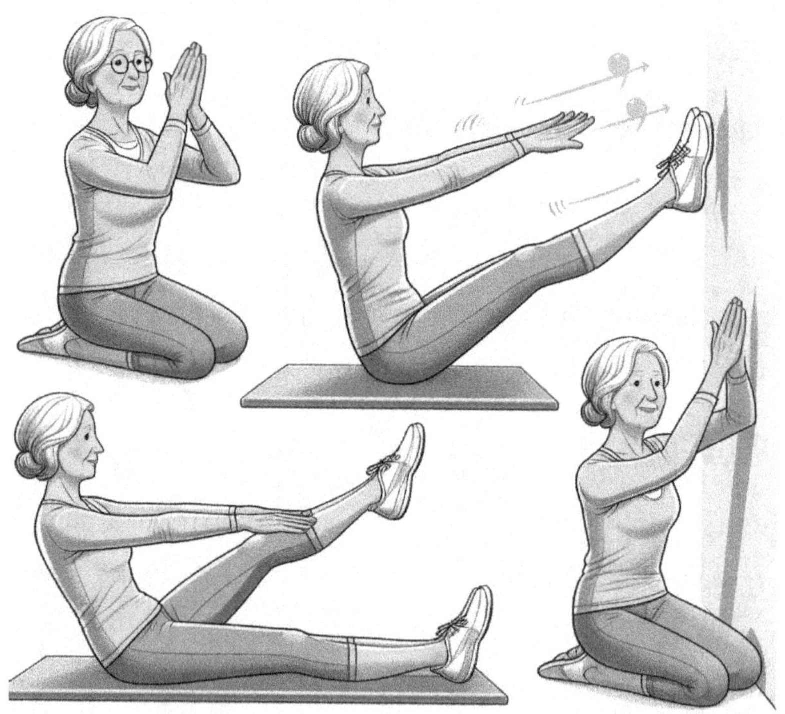

CHAPTER 5

Nutrition and Hydration for Active Seniors

Nutrition and hydration are critical factors in the health and performance of active seniors, especially those who engage in low-impact aerobic activities. A well-balanced diet and enough of fluids are crucial for feeding the body, speeding up recovery, and maintaining general health. Understanding how to fuel their bodies adequately is critical for seniors to maintain an active lifestyle, since they may have particular dietary demands and hydration difficulties.

Nutrition for Active Seniors.

A balanced diet for active seniors should contain items from all food categories, such as fruits and vegetables, whole grains, lean proteins, and healthy fats. This variety guarantees a proper amount of vitamins, minerals, and nutrients required for energy, muscle repair, and general health.

Proteins are essential for muscle repair and development. Lean meats, poultry, fish, eggs, dairy products, legumes, and nuts are all potential sources.

Carbohydrates are the body's principal energy source. Choose complex carbs like whole grains, fruits, and vegetables, which also include fiber and vital minerals.

Fats are necessary for energy and cell function. Focus on healthy fats from avocados, olive oil, almonds, and fatty seafood.

Vitamins and Minerals: Calcium and vitamin D are especially necessary for bone health, B vitamins for energy metabolism, and antioxidants for cellular repair.

Portion Control: As metabolic rates decline with age, portion control can help avoid weight gain and improve general health. Listening to your hunger cues and eating thoughtfully can help you maintain portion management.

Seniors are more likely to experience dehydration due to physiological changes that impair water conservation. Regular fluid intake is vital, especially during strenuous exercise.

Water is the greatest option for staying hydrated. Active seniors should strive to drink at least 8 glasses of water each day, with adjustments based on activity level, weather circumstances, and personal needs.

Electrolyte Balance: Drinking fluids containing electrolytes (sodium, potassium, magnesium) can assist maintain the body's electrolyte balance, which is essential for muscular performance and fluid retention during extended activity, particularly in hot weather.

Tips to Ensure Adequate Nutrition and Hydration

- Plan Meals: Planning meals and snacks around workouts can help seniors get the energy they need for exercise and the nutrients they need to recuperate. A modest, carbohydrate-rich snack before exercise can offer energy, and a protein-rich post-workout meal can help with muscle repair.

- Hydration Before, During, and After Exercise: Drink water before you begin exercising, take tiny sips throughout the activity to keep hydrated, and drink water afterward to restore any fluids lost via perspiration.

- Monitor Hydration Status: Pay attention to indicators of dehydration, such as thirst, dry mouth, decreased urine production, or dark urine. Seniors should not wait until they are thirsty to drink water, as thirst sensations might fade with age.

- speak Healthcare Providers: Before making large adjustments to diet or hydration practices, particularly for individuals with health concerns or using medicines, it is best to speak with a healthcare professional or a nutritionist to verify that the modifications support overall health and fitness objectives.

- Proper diet and hydration are essential components of a healthy lifestyle for active seniors. Seniors who focus on a balanced diet and proper hydration consumption can improve their exercise performance, promote recovery, and support their general health and well-being while engaging in low-impact aerobic activities.

Nutrition Basics for Seniors

Nutrition is critical to the health and well-being of seniors, particularly those who are physically active and participate in low-impact aerobic activities. Our bodies change as we get older, which can have an impact on how we assimilate nutrients, our metabolism, and our nutritional demands. Understanding the fundamentals of nutrition is critical for seniors in order to maintain energy levels, promote physical health, and improve overall quality of life. Here's a detailed guide to dietary essentials for seniors.

1. Energy requirements.

Seniors often require fewer calories than younger persons due to a natural fall in basal metabolic rate and lower levels of physical activity. Active seniors, particularly those who engage in regular low-impact exercise, may require more calories than their less active counterparts to fuel their activities and promote recuperation. To maintain a healthy weight and promote physical activity, calorie intake should be balanced with energy expenditure.

2) Macronutrients

Proteins are necessary for repairing and growing tissues, particularly muscles. Seniors must consume enough protein to keep muscular mass, aid in recovery from activity, and maintain immunological function. Good sources include lean meats, fish, dairy products, beans, and nuts.

Carbohydrates are the major source of energy for the body. Seniors should eat complex carbs like whole grains, vegetables, and fruits, which give long-term energy and critical nutrients.

Fats are necessary for nutrition absorption and cell function. Seniors should consume healthy fats, such as avocados, olive oil, almonds, and fatty fish, while avoiding saturated and trans fats.

3. Micro-nutrients

- Aging can impair the absorption of different vitamins and minerals, therefore seniors should choose nutrient-dense diets.

- Calcium and Vitamin D are essential for bone health and help prevent osteoporosis. Dairy products, fortified meals, leafy greens, and sunshine exposure are all good sources of vitamin D.

- Vitamin B12 is essential for nerve function and red blood cell production. As absorption declines with age, seniors may require fortified diets or supplements.

- Fiber is essential for intestinal health and reducing constipation. Found in fruits, vegetables, whole grains, and legumes.
- Antioxidants: Protect against oxidative stress and inflammation. Colorful fruits and vegetables, such as berries and leafy greens, are great suppliers.

4. **Hydration**.

Seniors are more susceptible to dehydration, which can impair physical performance, cognitive function, and general health. Drinking enough fluids, particularly water, throughout the day is critical. Active seniors may need to drink more fluids to compensate for sweat losses when exercising.

5. **Practical Diet Tips**

Meal Planning: Preparing balanced meals with a range of food types can assist ensure that nutritional requirements are satisfied.

Smart snacking: Choosing nutrient-dense snacks like fruits, vegetables, and whole grains may give energy and critical nutrients in between meals.

Supplementation: Supplements may be required to address particular nutritional demands, such as vitamin D or B12, but it is critical to speak with a healthcare physician before beginning any supplement plan.

6. Consulting with Professionals

Given the complexities of nutrition and individual health demands, engaging with a nutritionist or healthcare practitioner may give tailored counsel to ensure dietary choices support general health, fitness goals, and any medical issues.

Understanding and adopting these nutrition essentials can help seniors, particularly those who do low-impact aerobic activities, maintain an active, healthy lifestyle. Seniors can improve their overall health by concentrating on balanced, nutrient-dense meals and enough water.

Essential Nutrients and Vitamins

For seniors who engage in low-impact aerobic activities, ensuring enough nutritional and vitamin consumption is critical for preserving energy, promoting recovery, and guaranteeing general health. As we age, our bodies may demand new dietary considerations, making some nutrients even as crucial. Here's an in-depth look at the critical minerals and vitamins required for active seniors.

- Macronutrients include proteins, which aid in tissue healing, immunological function, and muscle mass maintenance (which decreases with age). Lean meats, fish, poultry, eggs, dairy products, legumes, and nuts are all excellent sources of protein. For seniors, eating a variety of protein sources throughout the day can help them maintain muscular strength and energy levels.

- Carbohydrates are the body's principal fuel source. Seniors should consume complex carbohydrates such as whole grains, vegetables, and fruits, which give long-term energy and are high in fiber, vitamins, and minerals. Fiber, in particular, is necessary for digestive health and can help avoid constipation, a frequent problem among older persons.

- Fats: Healthy fats are required for brain function, energy, and nutritional absorption, particularly vitamins A, D, E, and K. Avocados, olive oil, fatty fish (such as salmon and mackerel), almonds, and seeds all contain beneficial fats. Incorporating them into meals can improve cardiovascular health and cognitive function.

Micronutrients

- Vitamin D and Calcium: These nutrients work together to promote bone health, which is critical for preventing osteoporosis, a condition that older citizens are especially vulnerable to. Dairy products, leafy green vegetables, and fortified foods provide calcium, whereas fatty fish, egg yolks, fortified meals, and sunshine contain vitamin D. Given the difficulty of receiving enough vitamin D from diet and sunlight alone, some seniors may require supplements, as prescribed by a healthcare practitioner.

- Vitamin B12 absorption, which is required for nerve function as well as the creation of DNA and red blood cells, might decrease as people age. Meat, fish, poultry, eggs, and fortified cereals are all potential sources. Seniors, particularly those following a vegetarian or vegan diet, may need to regularly check their B12 intake, perhaps necessitating supplementation.

- Antioxidants: Vitamins A, C, and E, as well as selenium, act as antioxidants, protecting the body from oxidative stress, which may lead to chronic illnesses and aging. A diet high in fruits, vegetables, nuts, and seeds can supply a variety of antioxidants that promote general health.

- Potassium is essential for cell function, nerve signaling, and fluid equilibrium. It can also assist counterbalance the effects of salt on blood pressure. Bananas, potatoes, spinach, and beans are all potential sources.

- Omega-3 Fatty Acids: Fatty fish, flaxseeds, chia seeds, and walnuts contain omega-3 fatty acids, which are beneficial to heart health. These fats are essential for cognitive function and may aid in reducing inflammation throughout the body.

Hydration

Adequate hydration is necessary for many biological activities, including digestion, food absorption, and muscular activity. Water is the greatest option for staying hydrated, although herbal teas and broths can also help with regular fluid consumption. Seniors should be aware of their hydration levels because the sense of thirst may reduce with age.

Adding Nutrients to the Diet

Creating balanced meals that contain a range of food categories is the most effective strategy to meet all of your nutritional needs. For seniors, particularly those who participate in low-impact aerobic activities, timing protein and carbohydrate consumption around exercise sessions can help fuel workouts and aid in recuperation.

Focusing on these critical minerals and vitamins can help active seniors sustain their physical activity, improve recuperation, and preserve general health and well-being, all of which contribute to a bright, active existence.

Meal Planning and Preparation

Meal planning and preparation are essential skills for seniors, particularly those who engage in low-impact cardio activities, since they help assure a well-balanced diet that promotes physical activity and general health. Seniors may ensure that they obtain enough nutrition to power their workouts and recuperate appropriately by planning their meals ahead of time. Here's a guide to successful meal planning and preparation:

Step 1: Assessing Nutritional Needs

First, determine your nutritional requirements depending on your exercise level, health status, and dietary limitations. This will help guide your food planning. For example, active seniors may require additional protein to aid in muscle regeneration and nutritious carbs for energy.

Step 2: Set Clear Goals.

Determine what you hope to achieve with your eating plan. Goals may include increasing energy levels, losing weight, or ensuring enough consumption of certain nutrients such as calcium for bone health or fiber for intestinal wellness.

Step 3: Gather recipes.

Collect recipes that meet your dietary demands and personal taste preferences. Choose meals that are well-balanced and include a range of dietary categories, such as proteins, whole grains, vegetables, fruits, and healthy fats. Consider recipes that may be simply adapted to your preferences or dietary requirements.

Step 4: Make a Meal Schedule

Create a weekly meal plan that includes what you'll eat for breakfast, lunch, supper, and snacks. Balance your meals throughout the day to stay energized and avoid hunger. Include a variety of foods to guarantee a diverse range of nutrients.

Step 5: Create a Shopping List.

Create a grocery list based on your eating routine. To make your shopping trip more efficient, organize your list by store department (fruit, dairy, meats, and pantry goods). Stick to your list to prevent making impulsive purchases that do not fit into your eating plan.

Step 6: Schedule Preparation Time.

Set up dedicated time for meal preparation. This might include one huge session for the week's meals and smaller prep periods throughout the week for fresh things. To make the procedure pleasurable and easy, organize prep periods around your energy levels and schedule.

Step 7: Embrace batch cooking.

Prepare meals in batches to save time and keep healthful alternatives on hand. Cook big quantities of essentials such as rice, quinoa, or chicken breasts to be used in a variety of dishes throughout the week. Place portions in the refrigerator or freezer for quick access.

Step 8: Use Proper Storage.

Invest in high-quality storage containers to keep your cooked meals fresh. Label containers with the contents and date so you can keep track of what you have and save waste. Use clear containers to view what's within.

Step 9: Plan Your Snacks

Include nutritious snacks in your diet plan to keep your energy levels up in between meals. Prepare snack-sized quantities of fruits, veggies, almonds, or yogurt for convenient and healthful alternatives.

Step ten: Stay flexible.

While having a plan is crucial, you should also be flexible and prepared to adapt it based on how you feel, unexpected occurrences, or changes in appetite. Listen to your body and adjust your food plan accordingly to ensure that it continues to match your requirements and tastes.

By following these steps, seniors may establish a meal planning and preparation regimen that complements their low-impact aerobic activities and general health. This systematic approach to eating will help you maintain your energy levels, recover faster, and eat a balanced meal that contributes to a healthy, active lifestyle.

Hydration and Exercise

Hydration is critical for people's health and performance, especially seniors who engage in low-impact aerobic activities. Adequate fluid consumption is essential for sustaining basic processes, improving exercise performance, and promoting general health. Seniors' bodies lose water through perspiration while exercising, and this loss must be supplemented to avoid dehydration, which can have more serious consequences for older persons. Here's a detailed look at the necessity of water during exercise for seniors.

Understand the Importance of Hydration

Water is required for a variety of human processes, including maintaining body temperature, lubricating joints, and carrying nutrients. During activity, the body's requirement for water increases in order to cool itself through perspiration and maintain blood volume. Dehydration can impair physical performance, cause weariness, and raise the risk of heat-related disorders including heat stroke or heat exhaustion. Staying hydrated is especially important for seniors since the body's ability to save water declines with age, and thirst becomes less accurate as a hydration signal.

Identifying Dehydration Risks

Seniors are more likely to get dehydrated as a result of physiological changes that disrupt water balance. Reduced kidney function, chronic medical diseases (such as diabetes), and certain drugs can all contribute to increased dehydration risk. Symptoms of dehydration include dry mouth, weariness, dizziness, disorientation, and dark urine. Recognizing these symptoms early is critical to avoiding dehydration and its related hazards.

Seniors should drink water before exercising to be well hydrated. A basic advice is to consume around 17-20 ounces of water two to three hours before exercise.

During Exercise: Stay hydrated during your workout. Water is sufficient for hydration for low-impact exercises that last less than an hour. A excellent habit is to drink 7-10 ounces of water every 10-20 minutes while exercising.

Drinking water after exercise helps to replenish fluids lost during activity. This promotes healing and prepares the body for the next exercise. Consuming electrolyte-rich beverages or meals, such as potassium and salt, after prolonged exercise can help to restore what is lost via sweating.

Monitoring Hydration Levels.

Seniors can check their hydration levels by observing the color of their urine (light yellow indicates appropriate hydration) and being aware of thirst cues, which may be less apparent. Weighing oneself before and after exercise can also reveal fluid loss, with a loss of 1 pound indicating a fluid deficit of around 16 ounces.

Incorporating Hydration into Daily Life.

Integrating hydration practices into everyday routines can help seniors maintain a sufficient fluid intake. Carrying a water bottle, drinking water at regular intervals, and eating water-rich meals such as fruits and vegetables are all effective measures. It is also recommended to minimize your intake of caffeinated and alcoholic beverages, both of which can cause dehydration.

Personalizing Hydration Needs.

Individuals' hydration demands might vary greatly depending on body size, activity intensity, environment, and health problems. Seniors should tailor their hydration strategy to their own requirements, contacting healthcare specialists as needed, particularly if they have chronic diseases or take drugs that influence fluid balance.

Seniors who understand the importance of hydration in exercise and apply proper hydration measures can improve their exercise performance, recuperation, and general health during low-impact cardio exercises.

The Importance of Staying Hydrated

The significance of being hydrated cannot be emphasized, particularly for seniors who participate in low-impact aerobic activities. Water is required for almost all bodily functions, including temperature regulation, blood pressure maintenance, and cellular operations. Proper hydration is critical for active seniors because it improves physical performance, ensures exercise safety, and promotes overall health.

Hydration and Physical Performance.

Dehydration can drastically reduce physical performance. Even slight dehydration can impair endurance, cause tiredness, and weaken motivation. Water helps the body cool down through sweating, and dehydration can cause overheating and heat-related disorders, especially during heavy activity or in hot weather. Staying hydrated is critical for elderly who may have difficulty regulating body temperature.

Muscle and Joint Health.

Adequate hydration is essential for good muscle and joint health. Water lubricates joints, lowering the likelihood of discomfort and stiffness. It also helps to carry nutrients to the muscles, promoting recuperation and development. Proper hydration helps to prevent muscular cramps, which are a typical occurrence during exercise and can be aggravated by dehydration.

Cardiovascular Health

Hydration has a direct influence on cardiovascular function. When the body is dehydrated, blood volume falls, resulting in thicker blood and an increased heart rate. This causes additional pressure on the heart, making physical exertion more difficult. Staying hydrated supports normal blood volume and heart function, allowing for more effective blood flow and nutrition delivery throughout the body.

Cognitive Function and Mood

Hydration is also important for cognitive function and mood. Dehydration can impair focus, memory, and alertness, limiting an individual's ability to exercise and do everyday tasks. Furthermore, dehydration has been related to increased anxiety and weariness, whereas proper hydration can boost mood and energy levels.

Digestive Health and Nutritional Absorption

Water is essential for digestive health, helping to digest meals and absorb nutrients. It aids in the absorption of vitamins, minerals, and other nutrients from diet. Furthermore, sufficient water promotes good bowel motions and reduces constipation, which is a typical issue among seniors.

Strategies to Stay Hydrated

- Given the significance of hydration, particularly for active seniors, establishing techniques to guarantee proper fluid intake is critical.

- Consistent Fluid Intake: Drink water throughout the day, not only when exercising. Carrying a water bottle might act as a regular reminder.

- Monitor Urine Color: The color of urine is a useful measure of hydration levels; pale yellow indicates sufficient hydration, whereas dark yellow indicates dehydration.

- Incorporate Water-Rich Foods: Consuming fruits and vegetables with high water content, such as cucumbers, oranges, and watermelons, will help with total fluid consumption.

- Limit Diuretics: Drinks like coffee and alcohol have diuretic properties and can lead to fluid loss. Drinking in moderation might help them stay hydrated.

Staying hydrated is essential for seniors who want to live an active lifestyle and get the most out of low-impact aerobic activities. Seniors who prioritize water can improve their exercise performance, safeguard their health, and overall quality of life.

Tips for Adequate Hydration

Adequate hydration is vital for everyone, but it is especially important for seniors, particularly those who exercise often. As we age, our bodies become less effective in conserving water and more prone to dehydration. This can have an impact not only on overall health, but also on exercise performance and recovery time. Here are some practical strategies for seniors to stay hydrated, particularly when doing low-impact aerobic activities.

Understand Your Individual Needs

Individuals' water requirements vary substantially depending on their weight, degree of physical activity, climate, and health problems. While the usual recommended is 8 glasses (64 ounces) of water per day, active seniors may require more to compensate for fluid loss from sweating during activity. Pay attention to your body and adapt your water intake based on your individual requirements and daily activity.

Start Your Day With Water

Start each day with a glass of water. Overnight, your body loses water via breathing and sweat. Starting your day with water can help restore these losses and get you hydrated for the day.

Carry a water bottle.

Keeping a water bottle on hand acts as a continual reminder to hydrate during the day. Choose a reusable bottle that is convenient to carry and drink from. If you're going for a stroll or to a fitness class, remember to bring your water bottle to keep hydrated before, during, and after the activity.

Drink before feeling thirsty.

Thirst is not usually the greatest predictor of hydration, particularly in seniors, because the sense of thirst fades with age. Instead of waiting until you feel thirsty, establish a habit of drinking water at regular intervals throughout the day.

Incorporate foods with high water content.

Hydration is not just dependent on water. Many fruits and vegetables contain a lot of water, which can help you stay hydrated. Watermelon, strawberries, cucumbers, and lettuce are great options. Incorporating these water-rich items into your diet can help give necessary vitamins and minerals.

Monitor the color of your urine.

The color of your urine is a good measure of your hydration level. Pale, straw-colored pee indicates enough hydration, but dark yellow or amber-colored urine implies you should drink more water.

Limit caffeine and alcoholic beverages.

Caffeine and alcohol have diuretic properties, which might cause significant fluid loss. While you don't have to avoid these beverages totally, it's best to eat them in moderation and compensate with more water intake.

Use technology.

There are various applications available to help you track your water intake and remember to drink throughout the day.

Utilizing technology can help you accomplish your hydration objectives.

Listen to your body.

Pay attention to indicators of dehydration, such as dry mouth, fatigue, dizziness, and headaches. If you have any of these symptoms, drink more fluids.

Customize Your Hydration Strategy.

Hydration requirements might vary depending on the weather, your activity level, and your health state. In warmer weather or during strenuous activity sessions, you may require more fluids than normal. Similarly, if you're recovering from an illness or surgery, your fluid requirements may increase.

Seniors who follow these hydration guidelines can increase their exercise performance, recuperation time, and general health. Staying hydrated is a simple yet efficient strategy to preserve energy and lead an active lifestyle.

CHAPTER 6

Staying Motivated and Setting Goals

Staying motivated and having realistic objectives are critical components of a successful fitness journey, particularly for seniors who perform low-impact cardio activities. Motivation might fade as we age for a variety of reasons, including health difficulties, lifestyle changes, and a lack of rapid results. Setting attainable objectives and finding strategies to keep motivated can help seniors overcome these obstacles, allowing them to continue reaping the advantages of an active lifestyle. Here's how seniors may stay motivated and establish objectives for their low-impact cardio workouts:

Understanding Motivation

Motivation is very individualized and may be impacted by a variety of internal and external influences. Seniors may be motivated to exercise for a variety of reasons, including improving their health, increasing their mobility, maintaining their independence, or socializing. Identifying what motivates you is the first step toward developing and retaining motivation.

Setting SMART goals.

- Goals give direction and purpose, which helps you stay focused and motivated. SMART objectives (Specific, Measurable, Achievable, Relevant, and Time-bound) can be very effective:

- Specific: Clearly state what you aim to accomplish. Instead than "get fit," try "walk 30 minutes per day, five days a week."

- Measurable: Make sure your objective can be recorded, such as the length of exercise or the distance traveled.

- Achievable: Your objective should be tough but feasible based on your present physical condition and lifestyle.

- Relevant: Select objectives that are relevant and significant to you, and that are consistent with your health requirements and interests.

- Time-bound: Establish a deadline for completing your objective to keep you focused and motivated.

Find Your Why

Understanding why you want to be active may be a strong incentive. Whether it's spending time with grandkids, traveling, or simply enjoying a better quality of life, keep your motivations in mind.

Building a Support System

Surround yourself with supportive friends, family, or fellow fitness fanatics who will encourage your efforts. Joining a group fitness class or finding a workout companion might help you feel more connected and accountable.

Celebrating Milestones

Recognize and appreciate your accomplishments, no matter how minor. Achieving a goal or milestone may provide a substantial motivating boost. Non-food incentives might be a new book, a soothing bath, or new fitness gear.

Keeping it enjoyable

Choose things that you like to make exercise feel like a joyful part of your day rather than a chore. Changing up your routine might help to minimize boredom and keep training interesting.

Educate yourself.

Learning about the advantages of exercise and how they improve your health may be inspiring. Knowledge may help you make better decisions regarding your workout program.

Adjusting Goals As Needed

Prepare to adapt your goals depending on bodily input, changes in health state, or changes in interest. Flexibility can help you remain interested and motivated in the long run.

Visualizing Success.

Visualization methods, or visualizing oneself attaining your goals, may boost motivation and confidence. To encourage action, see yourself living an active, healthy lifestyle.

Staying motivated and establishing reasonable objectives are critical for seniors to continue reaping the benefits of low-impact cardio exercises. Seniors may maintain an active and meaningful lifestyle by knowing what motivates them, making realistic goals, and finding joy in their fitness journey.

SMART Goals for Fitness

SMART objectives are an effective strategy for improving fitness outcomes, particularly for seniors who perform low-impact cardio activities. SMART, which stands for Specific, Measurable, Achievable, Relevant, and Time-bound, is a framework for establishing clear and realistic goals. Applying SMART objectives to fitness can assist seniors in developing a focused and effective exercise plan, boosting motivation, measuring progress, and, ultimately, attaining greater health and wellness. Here's how to use SMART objectives to a workout routine for seniors:

Clear and defined goals are essential to minimize uncertainty and accomplish desired outcomes. Rather of a broad objective like "get in shape," a specialized goal might include the sort of exercise, length, and frequency. Let's say, for instance, "Walk for 30 minutes around the neighborhood every morning before breakfast." This clarity allows us to better focus our efforts and resources.

Measurable

A goal must be quantifiable in order to measure progress and determine when it has been reached. Numbers, such as distance, time, or frequency, enable objective measurement. For example, "Increase my walking distance to 2 miles per day" offers a concrete goal to strive for and measure against.

Achievable

While objectives should be difficult, they must also be realistic and achievable given present physical abilities and constraints. Setting an achievable objective considers elements such as baseline fitness levels, health issues, and lifestyle. A senior's feasible objective may be, "Attend two water aerobics classes per week," which is tough but doable with careful planning.

Relevant

The aim should be relevant to the individual's health requirements, interests, and life priorities. Relevance guarantees that the aim is worthwhile and compelling. For a senior who likes social activities, an appropriate objective may be to "join a senior walking group that meets twice a week." This is consistent with both fitness and social interaction aims.

Time-bound

Setting a time limit for a goal instills urgency and helps you stay focused. A time-bound objective has a deadline, which can encourage action and help prioritize activities. over example, "Walk 30 minutes per day, 5 days a week, for the next three months." This not only describes what has to be done, but also establishes a timetable for doing it.

SMART Goals for Senior Fitness

1. Assessment: Begin by examining your current fitness level, health status, and hobbies. This information will help you develop clear, attainable objectives.

2. Planning: Using the SMART criteria, create objectives that are matched to your fitness level and interests. For example, if flexibility is an issue, a particular objective can be, "Perform a 15-minute yoga session every morning to improve flexibility."

3. Tracking: Keep a journal or utilize applications to monitor your progress toward your goals. As you reach your objectives or your fitness levels change, evaluate and revise them on a regular basis.

4. Adjusting: Be prepared to change your goals as necessary. Flexibility is essential for retaining motivation and success,

particularly if you experience health changes or discover new activities that you like.

5. Seeking Support: Discuss your goals with friends, family, or fitness instructors who may provide encouragement, support, and accountability.

Setting SMART fitness objectives allows seniors to approach their low-impact cardio activities with a well-structured plan. This rigorous approach can result in increased motivation, continuous development, and, eventually, the adoption of a healthier, more active lifestyle.

Overcoming Challenges

Starting or sustaining a low-impact aerobic fitness plan as a senior presents distinct hurdles. These can include physical restrictions and health difficulties, as well as motivational and logistical challenges. However, overcoming these obstacles is crucial for seniors to continue receiving the multiple health advantages of regular exercise, such as better cardiovascular health, increased mobility, and improved mental well-being. Here are some tips for overcoming frequent problems in low-impact cardio routines for seniors.

Addressing Physical Limitations.

- Adapt workouts: One of the most effective strategies to deal with physical limits is to modify workouts to better suit one's ability. For example, if standing workouts are difficult, consider seated versions or water aerobics to relieve joint tension. Working with a physical therapist or a trained fitness expert can result in tailored modifications.

- Begin with low-intensity workouts and gradually increase the time and intensity to allow the body to acclimate without becoming overwhelmed. This progressive approach lowers the likelihood of damage and makes the workout more bearable.

Managing Health Concerns

- Consult healthcare providers. Before beginning any new fitness plan, seniors should contact with their healthcare specialists, particularly if they have chronic diseases such as heart disease, diabetes, or arthritis. This ensures that the chosen activities are both safe and beneficial.

- Monitor Health: It is critical to pay close attention to the effects of exercise on one's health and alter actions accordingly. If a certain workout causes discomfort or exacerbates health problems, it may be important to attempt other activities or change the current regimen.

Staying motivated

- Set Realistic objectives: Setting attainable, detailed objectives may create a sense of direction and success, increasing motivation. Celebrating tiny victories along the road can also boost perseverance.

- Find Fun Activities: Exercising does not have to be tedious. Finding things that you like makes it simpler to stay engaged. Whether it's dancing, swimming, or wandering in nature, partaking in enjoyable workouts may boost motivation greatly.

- Join fitness clubs or courses to gain social support, making exercises more pleasurable and less alienating. Sharing objectives with friends and family members who may give support is also important.

Navigating Logistics Issues

- Create a Convenient Routine Creating an exercise program that is easy to incorporate into your everyday life might help to alleviate logistical issues. This might entail picking workouts that can be done at home or finding a gym that is nearby and easily accessible.

- Utilize Resources: Taking advantage of local community resources, such as senior centers or parks, may provide convenient and often free ways to keep active. Many cities provide programs exclusively for elders.

Handling Setbacks

- Be Flexible: Adaptability is essential while dealing with setbacks. Illness, injury, or personal demands may all disrupt fitness schedules. Being willing to change your plan, such as modifying the type or intensity of exercise, might aid in maintaining progress.

- Prioritize recuperation: If a setback occurs as a result of an injury or sickness, recuperation must come first. This might include rest, physical therapy, or reduced routines that allow the body to recuperate while remaining as active as possible.

- Seek Professional Advice: When faced with a dilemma, speaking with fitness professionals, healthcare specialists, or physical therapists can give helpful insights and solutions.

Overcoming the difficulties connected with low-impact cardio activities for seniors takes a combination of flexibility, effort, and assistance. Seniors can continue to benefit from an active lifestyle by addressing physical limits, managing health concerns, keeping motivated, navigating logistical obstacles, and dealing with setbacks in a positive and proactive manner, so improving their overall health and quality of life.

Dealing with Setbacks

Setbacks are an unavoidable part of any fitness journey, especially for seniors who perform low-impact cardio routines. These might include everything from health problems and injuries to low motivation and logistical challenges. How seniors adapt to and deal with these setbacks is critical to their physical activity and general well-being. Here's a complete approach on dealing with setbacks in senior fitness.

Acknowledge and accept.

The first step in dealing with a setback is to accept it without passing judgment. Accepting that setbacks are a normal part of the process, whether they are caused by an accident, a health issue flare-up, or a loss of enthusiasm, is critical. It is critical not to allow guilt or irritation to take control, since these emotions can impede rehabilitation and growth.

Assess and understand.

Take the time to examine the setback and determine its reasons. Is it the result of overexertion, poor recuperation, an associated health condition, or even external stressors? Identifying the fundamental cause will help you develop an effective reaction strategy and avoid such setbacks in the future.

Consult Healthcare Professionals.

When setbacks include injuries or health difficulties, working with healthcare specialists is critical. They can provide an accurate diagnosis, prescribe a treatment plan, and advise on when and how to safely resume physical activity. This phase is critical for ensuring that any return to activity is useful rather than harmful to rehabilitation.

Adjust your fitness plan.

Adjust your workout regimen based on professional guidance and your own unique assessment. This might include lowering the intensity or duration of exercises, moving to safer or more realistic kinds of exercise, or even taking a total break to allow for recovery. Flexibility in your approach to exercise is essential for overcoming setbacks.

Focus on What You Can Do.

Instead than concentrating on the restrictions presented by the setback, consider what you can still do. For example, if an injury prohibits you from walking, you may still be able to do sitting strength exercises or light stretching. Maintaining an active mentality might help you maintain your physical and mental health during rehabilitation.

Set new and realistic goals.

Setbacks frequently involve modifying your fitness objectives. Set fresh, realistic goals that reflect your present position. These objectives should be attainable and inspiring, providing as a guide for your modified training regimen. Remember to apply the SMART criteria (Specific, Measurable, Achievable, Relevant, and Time-bound) while developing goals.

Seek support.

Asking for help might make dealing with setbacks easier. This might be joining a support group for others facing similar issues, connecting with a fitness community, or simply sharing your experiences with friends and family. Support networks may offer support, guidance, and inspiration.

Be patient and persistent.

Patience is essential while dealing with setbacks. Recovery and growth might take time, so it's crucial to follow your body's pace. Persist in your attempts to keep active within your existing abilities, and be willing to progressively increase your activity level as you recuperate.

Reflect and learn.

Finally, turn setbacks into learning opportunities. Consider what happened, how you reacted with it, and what you could do differently in the future. This reflection might help you build resilience and prepare for future problems.

Dealing with setbacks effectively requires a combination of acceptance, adaptability, and active participation in rehabilitation. Seniors may negotiate setbacks in their low-impact cardio workout routines by taking a flexible approach to fitness, obtaining expert counsel, and using support networks, allowing them to sustain their physical activity and contribute to their long-term health and wellbeing.

Staying Positive and Resilient

Staying optimistic and resilient in the face of adversity is critical for seniors who participate in low-impact aerobic programs. The quest to maintain an active lifestyle in older age can be fraught with ups and downs. Adjusting to physical restrictions, dealing with health setbacks, or just finding the drive to continue active may all put a strain on one's commitment. However, establishing a positive mentality and resilience can greatly improve one's capacity to overcome these obstacles and get the advantages of regular exercise. Here's how elders may remain optimistic and resilient:

cultivate a growth mindset.

Adopting a growth mindset, or the concept that talents and skills can be developed through devotion and hard effort, is essential for resilience. Rather than perceiving problems as insurmountable, consider them chances to learn and grow. Celebrate tiny successes and progress, no matter how gradual, since they lead to long-term success.

Set realistic expectations.

Setting reasonable expectations for what you can do with your workout program is critical. Recognize and respect your body's limitations, and be aware that growth in physical fitness, particularly for seniors, can be sluggish and non-linear. Adjusting expectations to reflect realistic outcomes helps you stay motivated and satisfied with your efforts.

Focus on What You Can Control.

Focusing on parts of your fitness journey that you have control over, such as your attitude, effort, and how you respond to setbacks, may help you feel empowered and resilient. While you may not be able to control some health conditions or the aging process, you can adjust your exercises, regulate your nutrition, and stay devoted to your goals.

Practice gratitude.

Practicing thankfulness by noticing and appreciating the good parts of your life and fitness journey might help you feel better overall. Regularly focusing on what you're grateful for, such as your ability to move, the support of friends and family, or the progress you've made, can help you change your emphasis away from obstacles and toward optimism.

Create a supportive community.

Surrounding yourself with a supportive group of friends, family, or fellow fitness fanatics that inspire and uplift you may have a huge impact on your optimism and resilience. Participating in group exercise courses or joining fitness programs for seniors may provide social support, accountability, and a feeling of community.

Embrace self-compassion

Be nice and sympathetic to oneself, particularly during stressful times. Understand that setbacks are a natural part of the process and do not represent your merit or effort. Treat yourself with the same compassion and understanding that you would show a friend in a similar position.

Stay adaptable and open to change.

Being willing to change your workout program in response to new talents or interests demonstrates resilience. Flexibility enables you to continue engaging in physical activity in a way that is appropriate for your present condition, ensuring that you can remain active and get the advantages of exercise.

Engage in positive self-talk

The way you communicate to yourself has a huge influence on your thinking and resilience. Positive affirmations and constructive self-talk can help replace negative or self-defeating ideas. Remind yourself of your strengths, prior triumphs, and the reasons you're determined to keep active.

Seek inspiration.

Look for tales about other seniors who have successfully maintained an active lifestyle or overcome comparable obstacles. These tales can provide you encouragement, inspiration, and practical advice for navigating your own fitness path.

Staying cheerful and resilient enables seniors to face the obstacles of leading an active lifestyle with grace and resolve. Seniors can benefit from low-impact cardio workouts by adopting a growth attitude, setting realistic goals, concentrating on controllable aspects, and using support networks, so improving their quality of life.

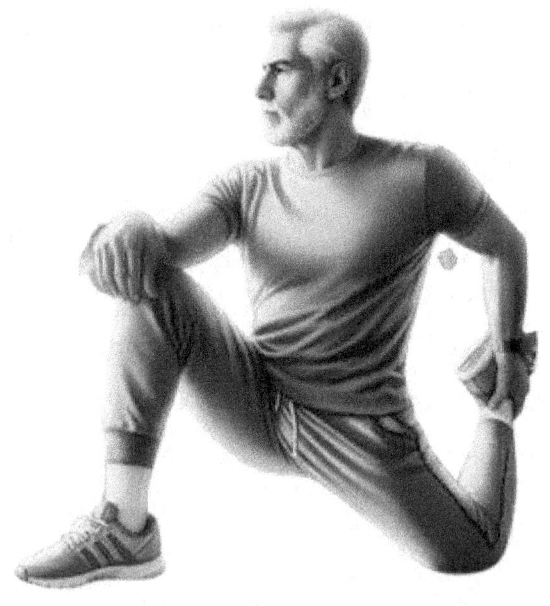

CONCLUSION

Starting a low-impact aerobic training regimen to improve one's health and energy is a respectable move, particularly for seniors. The "Low-Impact Cardio Workout for Seniors" guide is more than just a book; it's a companion who will lead you through every step of the trip, providing practical guidance, personalized workouts, and motivating insights intended exclusively for the unique requirements of older folks. It simplifies the process of remaining active, making it more accessible, pleasant, and, most importantly, safe for seniors looking to improve their quality of life.

As you examine the actions to improve your health and well-being, keep this advice handy. It is designed with the belief that every senior has the opportunity to live a more active, healthier, and satisfying life, regardless of current fitness levels or previous exercise experiences. By including low-impact cardio activities into your daily routine, you not only improve your physical fitness but also your mental health, enhance your energy levels, and nurture a stronger feeling of independence.

We cordially welcome you to use this chance to better your life. **Buy your copy of "Low-Impact Cardio Workout for Seniors" today** and take the first step toward a healthier, more vibrant future. Your road to better fitness and well-being begins here, with each page of this book designed with your requirements in mind.

We'd appreciate it if you could share your ideas and experiences after using this complete guide. Your candid evaluation might inspire other elders to begin their fitness journeys, spreading the message of health and vitality far and wide. By sharing your experience, you become a source of inspiration, demonstrating that it is never too late to make great changes in one's life.

Your input not only recognizes your accomplishments, but also helps to build a community of active, health-conscious seniors. **Let us work together to create a future in which all seniors have the tools and confidence to live an active and satisfying life. Join us by grabbing your book and, after enjoying the advantages, leaving an honest review of "Low-Impact Cardio Workout for Seniors."**

www.ingramcontent.com/pod-product-compliance
Lightning Source LLC
Chambersburg PA
CBHW050821260726